Disclaimer Notice:

Please note the information contained within this document is for educational and entertainment purposes only. All effort has been executed to present accurate, up to date, reliable, complete information. No warranties of any kind are declared or implied. Readers acknowledge that the author is not engaging in the rendering of legal, financial, medical or professional advice. The content within this book has been derived from various sources. Please consult a licensed professional before attempting any techniques outlined in this book.

By reading this document, the reader agrees that under no circumstances is the author responsible for any losses, direct or indirect, that are incurred as a result of the use of information contained within this document, including, but not limited to, errors, omissions, or inaccuracies.

Table of Contents

Sex Positions for Couples

Learn the Best Positions to Unleash Your Sexual Energy and Transform Your Sex Life. Enjoy Spectacular Experiences of Pleasure Using Tantric Techniques and Special Tips

by

Marissa Foster and Christian Murray

Introduction

A new relationship is a journey into a world of commitment, goals, and intimacy. As you begin to bond with a new partner, you may want to explore life together, and this includes lovemaking and the principles of pleasure. This book will provide you with a guide into the basics of sex and intimacy so that you develop a strong, healthy relationship with your partner. Before you engage in a variety of sexual activities, it is important to communicate and discover everything you both have in common. This book gives you the tools to be open with your partner and to develop a deep understanding and appreciation for all the pleasure you can explore and enjoy together.Intimacy is an important part of every relationship. Getting to know your partner and connecting with them on a deeper level through communication and affection can go a long way to ensuring a relationship grows into a strong and resilient love that can last for decades. While this book primarily focuses on intimacy in new couples, anyone in any type of relationship can apply the principles and suggestions offered here.

Intimacy evolves over time, from intense and frequent to more routine and sometimes infrequent. For this reason, more effort and creativity should be placed, from increasing the spontaneity in your marriage or relationship to creating a surprise for your partner with a new activity or idea.

If you are with a new partner or spouse, it may take time to become comfortable and well acquainted with them. Every situation is different. Some couples progress quickly, while others take their relationship slowly. In every personal relationship, there needs to develop a strong sense of trust and open communication first, as these both serve as a solid foundation for a close, loving bond. When the power of trust and communication is underestimated, challenges and misunderstandings could arise, often leading to unintended difficulties and hurt. Most, if not all, future problems can be averted with a strong desire to communicate and understand the other person's priorities.

Becoming familiar and comfortable with intimacy early in the relationship means getting to know your partner by spending time with them and discussing a wide variety of topics, including sex and lovemaking practices. Some people with little or no sexual experience may find this difficult at first, though it can get much easier over time with practice and familiarity.

Chapter 1: Your Partner and Intimacy

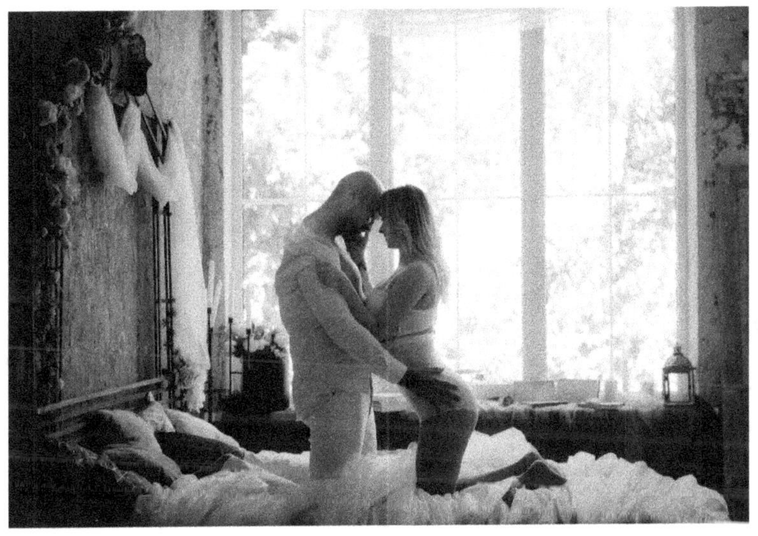

Finding a compatible partner is an incredible journey that can help us learn a lot about ourselves and what we want and need in life. For some people, there are social obstacles that can prevent them from fully engaging with others and bonding with them. In the beginning stages of a relationship, a euphoric sense of excitement and strong arousal builds, and this can be difficult to navigate for some people. There are many reasons why people hesitate to initiate sex or intimacy, and this can become a hurdle, especially in the early stages of the relationship.

Shyness in the bedroom is not an uncommon experience, but most people do not discuss their shyness associated with this situation as it is personal in nature. Most people will often think they are the only ones who feel that way and no one else when, in reality, this is not true, as most people have felt shy at least on one occasion.

The first step to overcoming shyness is to understand its causes and explore them further. These may include cultural and societal expectations, which vary in different regions around the world. It is also helpful to find out whether the roles of men and women are traditional or progressive. There is also the individual perspective, which involves how we see ourselves and how we think others view us, versus the reality.

Common Reasons for Intimacy Challenges

1. *Many women are uncomfortable with their physical bodies.* Because of this, they may avoid intimacy. In fact, close to 70 percent of women claim they are generally unhappy with their appearances and avoid intimacy for this reason. Men can experience this, too, but it appears to affect more women on average. There is a tremendous pressure to conform to a variety of beauty standards set by society, and anything outside of these standards is considered unacceptable or less.

Fortunately, there have been positive strides in recent years to embrace a variety of body shapes and sizes. The fashion industry is slowly transitioning toward highlighting more "curvy" or realistic body shapes that most women can relate to (Relationship Guide Review, 2019).

2. *Some people are afraid to initiate sex for fear of rejection.* This extends to both men and women. Even when people are interested in sex, they would rather not take their risk of being rejected. This results in them missing the chance of potentially developing a relationship that could otherwise be healthy and enjoyable. It is important to understand that rejection happens to everyone at some point or another. While it can feel personally hurtful, it is best not to take rejection negatively, as there are often reasons beyond what you may know and understand. Some people may have deep personal reservations about the idea of sex, possibly caused by a traumatic event in the past, making them respond negatively to it. Showing empathy, understanding, and acceptance is important in these circumstances.

3. Some communities follow traditional rules and practices regarding sex and intimate relationships. Because of this, many women and men are unable to adequately express their sexual desires or fantasies without scrutiny. Finding privacy may also be a challenge if family and community members are encouraged to chaperone or accompany couples during the early stages of dating.

4. Progressive societies that embrace a more open-minded approach to sex can invite more expectations from a partner. A person may develop a sense of inadequacy when they feel that their sexual experience does not measure up to their partner's standards. Some people are so caught up with making a good first impression, they forget to enjoy the person they are with and the relationship as a whole.

5. Finally, if you are young with little or no experience with sex, developing a relationship with a partner is a completely new territory. In a relationship, it takes a lot of time and communication to get to know each other well and feel comfortable being intimate.

Chapter 2: Sounds of Love

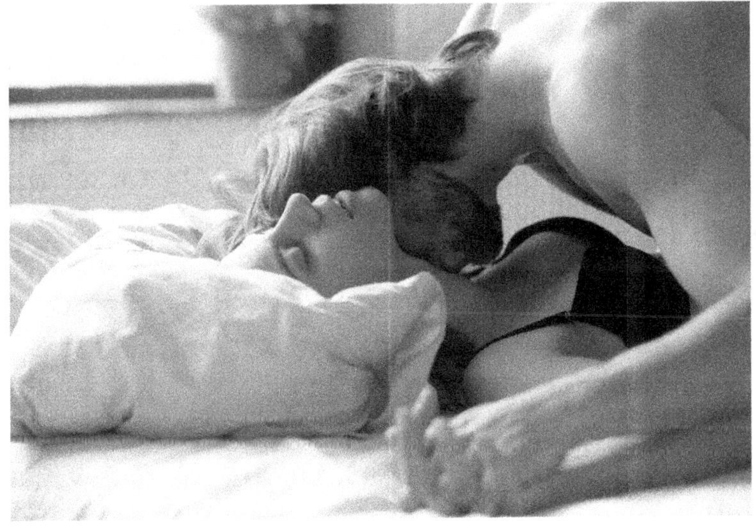

Whether we are aware or not, it is common for people to vocally express pleasure and emotions during lovemaking. During sex, there are subtle sounds that convey various messages, such as wanting more. Every person vocalizes differently. Some people make a lot of sounds in bed, while others tend to be quiet and less vocal. The sounds we produce during sex affect our performance and our experience with our partner.

How We Communicate During Sex

Usually, TV shows and films depict vocals during sex in an intense way, and they often highlight climatic sounds of arousal. However, there are far more subtle sounds, movements, and gestures that can give much more depth to your sexual experience.

Non-verbal cues can indicate what your partner wants during sex, from engaging further to initiating a new position. Furthermore, the various sounds we make, such as a groan or grunt, can enhance our pleasure.

Let us take for example a bird that is about to take flight.

It may chitter or vocalize its takeoff, do an embellished flapping of its wings, and extend its body. This behavior affects the bird's flying experience while also signaling to other birds that it is about to fly. This is similar to sex. When your lover makes grunts or groans during a lovemaking session, it means they are experiencing pleasure and letting you know about it! It might be subtle at first, and then it becomes more expressive. When you moan during lovemaking, it does not only give your partner an indication of your experience but also enhances your own sensation.

Vocals During Sex: What Do They Mean and What to Look For

How do we interpret the various sounds we make during sex? Some of the sounds we make are not initially made for the purpose of communicating but are more of a reaction to our own experience. The vocals we produce let our partners know what we want and how we feel during our interaction with them. The following are the different types of sounds and breathing that indicate various things.

Short, rapid breathing indicates a growing amount of excitement as arousal builds up during sex. Typically, this is the sound of pleasure as one partner begins to arouse their lover during sex. This usually occurs in the early stages, when initial foreplay begins or slips into a more intense exchange of touching, leading to sex.

Grunts and groans are usually sounds that occur during sex as a reaction to various techniques and movements, giving your partner an indication of how they are progressing. During lovemaking, we may not be able to explicitly say how we feel or direct our partners where to pleasure us, but when the reaction is a grunt or a groan, it essentially says, "Yes, right there, that's it." As the pleasure increases in intensity, progressing toward a climax, the moaning becomes louder, and we may clench our fists or contract our muscles.

Moans and other sounds that may indicate something completely different from pleasure (e.g., discomfort in a specific position) should cease.

In some cases, a partner directly indicates displeasure by saying, "Stop, I don't like that," or, "I need to change my position." However, there are also times when they only produce a sound that can be interpreted as the same statement so as not to interrupt the general flow or progression of the lovemaking.

As your partner or lover reaches orgasm, the sex noise intensifies as well, becoming louder and sharper, often accompanied by the contraction of muscles. It is the height of the experience, and it signals that your partner has achieved climax.

Vocals During Sex: How and When to Use Them

There's a lot to consider about sex and the way you vocalize with your partner during intimacy. When you vocalize our pleasure, it can boost the confidence of your partner. They may equate louder moans and quick breaths as increased pleasure and being closer to climax, and this is why many women, close to 80 percent, admit to faking an orgasm in this way at least half of the time.

This can cause confusion for couples who may not be keen on communicating openly about how they pleasure each other. It can mislead one to think they are adequately satisfying their partner when this is not accurate. On the other hand, when a partner is quiet and less expressive, it may prompt their lover to try harder and put more effort into lovemaking until they indicate their satisfaction.

How do we use vocals to communicate during sex to get the most out of pleasure and help our partner achieve their satisfaction as well? Be honest and responsive. Let your partner know when they are getting you closer to arousal. Vocals do not have to be overly loud or extreme. A few quick breaths and slight moans are enough to mean "Yes, that's it. Keep going." Or if a specific movement or action is not working, a simple "Let's try this instead" will do. You can also slightly adjust your body posture or position to change the method — that can work as well.

It is important to note that every couple communicates differently.

While being more explicit to one's comments and description works well for some, other people are less inclined to explain how they wish to be aroused, or they are less likely to ask their partner how best to satisfy them. Having a discreet yet direct conversation with your partner or lover can resolve a lot of mystery in your sex life and make it a more open and enjoyable experience. If you are not sure of how to ask, wait until you and your partner are alone and in a quiet, comfortable space where you can approach the topic. You will be pleasantly surprised by how well-received an open and candid discussion about sex can be!

Interesting Facts and Myths on the Sounds of Sex

There is a big difference between sexual activities depicted by the media and those in real life. Oftentimes, in adult films or mainstream television, couples having sex are shown in positions that make them appear glamorous or ideal physically, even when they do not normally appear this way in real life.

This extends to the sounds they make as well, where the louder and more vocal they become, the more aroused they are. This is especially grossly exaggerated in adult films, where the vocalization is overemphasized. What effect does this have on everyday couples? For people who regularly enjoy pornography, they may expect their partners to vocalize more than usual and achieve orgasm with little or no effort.

Some people think the louder the sounds, the better the orgasm. However, this is inaccurate in many situations. Some people are quiet during a climax. The success of orgasm is not measurable by the enthusiasm or crescendo of the sounds your partner makes. In fact, they may embellish things to give you the idea that they are reaching orgasm so that you will be satisfied in knowing you can bring them to that arousal. In reality, the loudest person can simply be expressing their pleasure despite being nowhere close to climax, and the quiet person may become less vocal as they reach orgasm. It purely depends on the individual, and it varies considerably from one person to another.

Talking dirty to your partner or teasing them with sexy whispers or comments is an exciting way to get them aroused. While this may seem stereotypical of film or sex scenes, talking dirty can definitely contribute in a positive way to sex and a couple's enjoyment of it. Imagine the reaction of your partner as you caress them with sexy words in the trace of a whisper. If you or your partner is new to this form of arousal, give it a try and gauge the response. Trying something at least once can be thrilling in itself and set the stage for more experimenting and fun later.

Chapter 3: Learn to Have Sex

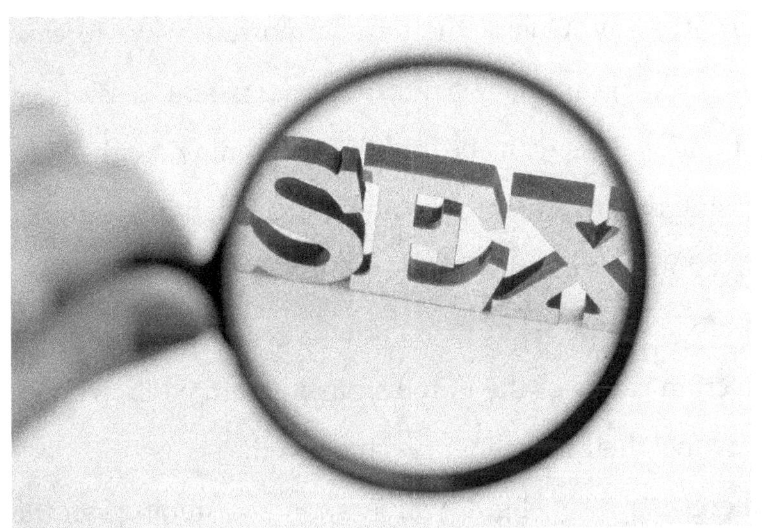

Having sex for the first time can be an exciting and nervous experience full of anticipation. It involves a wide range of emotions. Once you become familiar with sex, even if on a basic level, you will begin to learn what brings you and your partner pleasure. It could be through a certain touch or sensation. Try to see how your lover reacts when you kiss or touch them in a certain away. One of the most important ways to ease into sexual intimacy is through a gentle session of foreplay. This can be subtle, beginning with light kissing and touching, showing and exchanging signs of affection. During this phase, you may notice a decrease in anxiety and begin to experience signs of arousal. An erection is one of the initial signs in men, while women may feel their labia engorge and swell.

There may be slight wetness or moistening in the genital area, as well as heightened sensitivity to touch and sound. During this phase, the mutual attraction intensifies, which creates a transition to sex.

The Challenges of Sexual Education in Society

In many cultures and societies, sex education is considered taboo and avoided as much as possible. Even in countries where there is a more relaxed approach to the concept of sex and where it is introduced into the education system or discussed within the family, there still exists a gap between learning the fundamentals of biology and how to experience the pleasures of sexual activity. Sex education in most schools, for example, centers on the prevention of STIs (sexually transmitted infections), the concept of sexual arousal, and how the reproductive system works. In some progressive school systems, the curriculum has a broader spectrum of education to include all sexual orientations. These schools also have a more accepting approach to sexual and gender identity. However, there still exists a significant amount of resistance against a general openness to sexuality, and people are not generally taught how to enjoy and seek pleasure during sex.

Some family and marital arrangements have a heavy reliance on traditional practices that hold on to strict male and female roles. They place a more dominant role on men, with the expectation that women will always be sexually compliant and available even when there is no explicit consent. This power dynamic places men in a more commanding position where women's sexual needs and wants are suppressed.

On the other hand, men are expected to take on a traditional "leadership" role, which doesn't come with the goal of giving women pleasure or helping them achieve pleasure together as a couple. In relationships where there is both a lack of sexual education and mutual connection, sexual intimacy can be a major challenge, often done out of necessity and starting a family. Thus, it is less about pleasure and pleasing each other.

As some people break away from their traditional roles in marriage and intimate relationships, they realize there is much to learn from each other, especially on how to express their desires, bond with each other, and experience the joy of sex together.

While many people hold on to traditional views of marriage and sex, it is important to recognize the importance of learning the value of pleasure: how to please ourselves and our partners. This will only become easier for people once the stigma of sexual openness and communication fades away over time, allowing more discussion and direct communication about sex and how we can enjoy it.

Important Facts About Sex Everyone Should Know

Learning about sex goes beyond the basics of biology. It goes beyond responding to various cues and states of arousal. There are a lot of interesting facts to know about sex. If you are new to sex or less experienced, you will find that the early stages are a combination of learning from what you hear, read, and experience first-hand.

If you are more knowledgeable than your partner, you can provide more guidance. However, care should always be taken so that both of you feel comfortable and willing to engage.

The following important facts are vital and interesting, and they should be considered before you decide to engage with your partner.

1. Consent should be explicit

When it comes to sex, a simple "Yes, I want to make love" is not always the way we consent or agree to have sex.

When one partner initiates intimacy, the other may appear interested at first and then may hesitate later on. The reasons can vary, from changing their mind to simply not being interested in the moment. When there is the slightest doubt, it is important to establish whether consent is present, and make sure both of you are completely 100 percent willing without any reservations.

There should be explicit consent, which means you and your partner should be fully in agreement and enthusiastic about it.

2. *Sex is not going to be the same experience every time.*

Some sessions will be groundbreaking and exciting, leaving you wanting more. On other occasions, sex is less than thrilling and may not bring both or either partner to orgasm.

This can be a result of various things — e.g., personal trauma in life, stress from family or work, or simply not feeling completely engaged or aroused in the experience. This is perfectly normal. It would be unusual to have ideal sex each and every time, as this is unrealistic. Do not expect this to happen always. It is important to be realistic, and accept the fact that, on some occasions, the spark may not be present. Be patient, and you will find that the best experiences will return again.

3. *Long sessions of sex do not equate to better quality, and short, quick sex does not always have to be negative either.*

It really depends on the couple and the circumstances. For example, in the morning, a quick session of early sex may be brief but highly passionate and satisfying.

In fact, both lovers may be familiar enough with each other to bring about orgasm within a short time span, and then they go their separate ways for work and other daily activities.

A longer session in a rushed morning would not accommodate their schedule. On the other hand, a slower, deeper intimacy in the evening hours can be satisfying in a completely different way, allowing both partners to experience more of each other.

4. *Erection does not happen instantly every time, and when it does, it may occur when it is least expected.*

A man may find himself with an erection in the morning during a shower or as he's getting ready for breakfast. A woman, on the other hand, may feel aroused during regular activities, such as attending a conference or running errands.

When sex is initiated, it may take time to achieve an erection and natural arousal, even where both lovers are ready and excited to begin.

5. *Lubrication is good for everyone.*

It is wonderful how our bodies can create our own wetness, though it is best to add a bit of natural lubricant to your sexual encounter to avoid dryness and irritation later.

There are various brands to choose from. You can also choose a variety of flavors and/or scents. There is also a choice between a more sensitive and natural fluid versus a more standard one. Take time to shop around with your partner to determine which one works best for both of you.

6. *Moving from one position to another during sex is not always a simple task.*

It mainly depends on your flexibility. Try new poses or positions, and switch them up every now and then. Some moves are going to take some practice, even exercise, to get them just right.

Some positions may require your partner to lend you a hand, or you may need to help them steady their balance or ease slowly into a new pose. It may not look and feel glamorous, but it will be fun just the same!

7. Using protection is important, and knowing how to use it is vital.

Condoms are the most commonly used and preferred method of birth control and protection against STIs (sexually transmitted diseases). They are important early in the relationship. However, learning how to use a condom for the first time can be frustrating, and it often causes friction if not lubricated well. Condoms are not all created equally. Some brands may boast high sensitivity, while others are more durable and already lubricated, making it easier to put on. To avoid potential breakage and to ensure your experience is not spoiled, make sure you have a few condoms handy, just in case. Read the instructions carefully and take it slowly at first until you become used to the procedure.

Remember that your partner can be helpful and give you much-needed support and assistance to get your session underway. There are creative and fun ways of putting on a condom, and this can fit easily into foreplay, making the experience much more enjoyable.

8. *Sex is good for your health, and it is a form of exercise.*

The more often you engage, the more calories you will burn. It is great for the heart and your body in general. Sex itself is a euphoric experience, causing a release of endorphins in the body, which reduces the likelihood of depression, anxiety, and other disorders. The frequency of sex varies from one couple to another, and while it is often more often at the beginning of the relationship, a routine will eventually become established. Even if you are engaging twice a week, there are fantastic benefits to your health and well-being.

9. *Smoking can have a negative impact on your sex life.*

Not only is smoking bad for your health, but it is also associated with lower rates of arousal and a decline in the strength of an erection. It can also affect endurance, making it difficult for the smoker to last longer in the bedroom, especially where there are respiratory conditions involved.

If you currently smoke, consider quitting or taking steps to decrease the amount you use, as this will make a major improvement over time.

10. *Orgasm is not going to happen every time you have sex.*

You can have a hot and passionate session with your partner and not achieve a climax. Likewise, your partner can experience the same; it happens for both men and women. It can cause feelings of disappointment and insecurity. It is normal for this to occur sometimes, even between health-loving couples.

11. *The more you communicate, the better your sex life will be.*

Many people avoid talking about certain topics, including sex and intimacy.

When communication breaks down, it can lead to a lot of misunderstandings, hurt, and avoidance. Intimacy can eventually break down until it reaches the point where it is no longer a part of a couple's life.

Once this happens, it can lead to marital or relationship breakdown as well. Keeping the conversation alive is the best way to enjoy all that your relationship can provide.

There are many other facts about sex that you can learn in a variety of ways. One of the best ways to get familiar with your body and to engage with your partner is through open dialogue and discussion about a variety of concerns, including your fantasies and desires (Gordon, 2018).

Five Uncommon Facts That Can Improve Your Sex Life

Getting comfortable with your partner will not only help improve your sex life but will also give you the confidence to ask questions and better understand how you can mutually pleasure each other. Exploring various techniques and ideas and having an openness to doing so has a major impact on the success of your love life and how well it will develop over time. Couples who explore and communicate about sex without reservation tend to lead healthier, happier lives in general, not just in the bedroom.

There are a few unexpected ideas and facts that make a positive impact on your sex life. Some of these facts dispel myths about sex, giving us a different perspective on how to enjoy our love life. They also create a healthy outlook about sex and how we engage with our partner and ourselves.

1. The most sexual part of our body is our brain.

The onset of arousal and the creation of sexual fantasies begins here.

It is our mind that plays the most significant role in how we experience lovemaking and how we connect with our partner. Our perception (the signals our body and mind process and send throughout our body during foreplay and sex) sets the stage for a spectacular series of sensations. Alternatively, when our thoughts or impressions about a specific scenario are negative, it affects our body's response. For example, if we feel hesitant about pursuing a specific technique with our partner or lack trust in them for some reason, even the usual pleasurable event of lovemaking can be unenjoyable. This is because your mind isn't completely involved or relaxed for the experience. When we feel connected in mind and body, sex only gets better over time.

2. Women only orgasm 20 percent of the time during sex.

This is usually because some men believe women can achieve climax with vaginal sex alone, whereas this is not often the case.

In fact, most women need clitoral stimulation or oral sex to bring themselves to orgasm. In some positions, it is possible for both men and women to reach orgasm together, which can be incredibly pleasurable, though it can also take practice and time to achieve. It is also advantageous for couples to explore various forms of arousal, as well as positions that include oral sex. This will greatly increase the chances of orgasm for women and can help men as well.

3. Men also fake orgasms.

Women often admit to this, though men have been found to do this as well and often for the same reason: they want to please their partner or give the impression that they have been adequately satisfied. This may be a way for men to assure their partner that they are able to reach orgasm quickly and to convey confidence. For women, there are several reasons. Like men, they want to show their satisfaction or at least convince their partner of it.

Faking an orgasm gives the other person the satisfaction of being able to bring their partner to climax and, therefore, boosts their ego or confidence. The problem with this technique is dishonesty. Faking an experience you should want to enjoy is not giving you any real pleasure, while at the same time, it gives your partner the wrong impression of what works for you.

4. *Headaches and pain can often disappear or subside during sex.*

The popular excuse for declining sex, "Not tonight, I have a headache," is usually joked about as a means to avoid intimacy or skip sex. In reality, such an excuse could mean something more, especially if it is a recurring phrase (or something similar). There may be a hidden discomfort associated with sex that your partner may not feel like explaining, though they may be more direct and open with patience and understanding.

It is important to communicate to find out the real reasons for lack of intimacy and to gently approach the topic so as not to push or pressure your partner to explain everything, especially if there is (or are) reason(s) why they may not feel up to it (Hubby, 2017).

5. Many women masturbate, though they tend not to discuss it as freely or widely as men, mostly due to societal expectations and ideals.

Even where women have made great strides forward in freedom, including sexual expression and liberation, there are still items considered less favorable when broached by a woman than a man. Masturbation is one of these topics, as well as sex in general. However, this is changing, and women are becoming more vocal and expressive than ever. Masturbation, or self-pleasure, should never be a source of shame, whether you enjoy it for yourself or mutually with your partner (Carson, 2017).

Common Mistakes Men and Women Make During Sex

During the height of passion, where both lovers are completely mesmerized and connected, the slight error or misjudgment can thwart a good sexual experience completely. It happens even when we try our best, and knowing what can happen is one of the most important ways to avoid an embarrassing or uncomfortable situation that can impact the moment. Some mistakes we make are not sudden and unexpected; rather, they can become bad habits that repeat over time, dulling or killing the mood and atmosphere slowly over time or completely.

Avoid this and other pitfalls to keep your sex life amazing and mind-blowing. The following are common errors people often commit during sex. These are also some of the worst culprits of a declining sex life:

1. Skipping foreplay completely.

This means no foreplay at all, not even for a minute.

On average, foreplay occurs for about 10 or 15 minutes, and most men and women enjoy it more than they admit. Sometimes a quick session can mean less preparation time and more spontaneity, though this should not include leaving foreplay out of the picture completely. In fact, it should begin with foreplay and last at least for a couple of minutes. This stage is crucial in getting your partner aroused and ready for action. You will find that it benefits yourself as well, and the mutual affection grows together, setting the stage for a solid and enjoyable session of lovemaking, whether it is a quick play or a long and passionate session.

2. Poor hygiene.

This is a complete turn-off and can stop intimacy in its tracks. A little body odor or sweat after a trip to the gym or long cycling trip is natural and can actually be a turn-on, though a lack of proper hygiene on a recurring basis will often stop sexual attraction, especially if it becomes a habit. Taking good care of your body and how you treat yourself does not need to include fancy perfumes and body sprays.

Your natural scent is a part of the attraction, and with proper hygiene, your sex life will only get better.

3. Focusing on perfection.

Do not look in the mirror during sex and expect your body and your partner's to resemble a glamorous sex scene on television or film. You are not having sex to impress but to have fun and enjoy intimacy with your partner. Focusing too much on how to look better and appeal more to your partner may seem reasonable; we all want to look our best and get the most out of lovemaking. However, it can become unreasonably obsessive. Some people become so saturated in the way they look, even when their partner is happy with them as they are, that the pursuit of perfection can actually harm their marriage and sexual relations. Obsessing too much on your flaws takes the focus away from your partner and enjoying each other.

4. Talking about ex-partners or ex-spouses.

At some point in a relationship, the subject will arise, and that is expected.

However, it should not become a focal part of a conversation, especially where sex is involved. It is one of the top ways to turn off your partner and disengage. When you or your partner are in a heightened state of arousal, there's nothing worse than hearing about someone's ex-partner and how they employed certain sexual techniques in the bedroom. This will only give the impression that you are not interested in your partner, even where this is not the case at all. It can appear that by bringing up your ex, you are making a comparison between them, which can cause insecurity, even jealousy. Always choose your words carefully, and avoid discussion about past lovers, as they are no longer relevant.

5. Talking too much during sex.

This can be a turn-off, unless it is part of the act, such as sweet whispers and/or dirty talking, which can be deeply arousing and fun. Talking about unrelated matters, such as work, other people, and household matters, can dull the experience during sex.

This can happen if at least one partner becomes bored, and this can occur when sexual intimacy becomes routine or in a rut and no longer the fun, eventful activity it once was. If this becomes an issue, make it a point to try new and exciting positions. Play scenarios and techniques, many of which are covered in this book! (REL Rules, n.d.).

Chapter 4: The Different Types of Positions

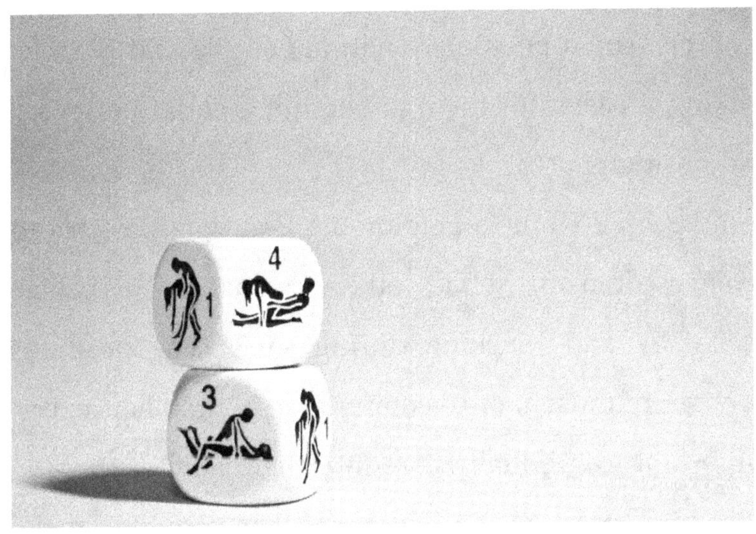

When people think of positions during sex, they may consider the most popular and common options that are often seen in films and TV shows. The missionary, doggy-style, and 69 positions are among the most discussed ones. Other widely known styles are the cowgirl style, reverse cowgirl style, and spooning. Trying new positions can be both fun and stressful, depending on how open and relaxed you feel. For example, some people are naturally agile and flexible, making it easier for them to attempt a variety of poses and positions.

Some people want to employ the best way possible to achieve orgasm, while others want to maximize sensuality and touching during sex. Some positions may seem unusual or uncomfortable at first; hence, it is important to gradually ease into them so that they do not cause pain or muscle strain that can hinder the experience.

New Positions to Try for a Better Experience

Some people are eager to try anything new that may bring a new layer of excitement to their sex life, and changing positions during sex can be one major way to achieve this. In fact, you can change positions and angles several times during one session of lovemaking. Don't be afraid to initiate a change in perspective or direction. If you are used to taking direction, making the suggestion for a change may come as a pleasant surprise to your partner. Aside from the common positions that we often see portrayed on screen, there are many interesting styles and variations to try.

The Lotus Position

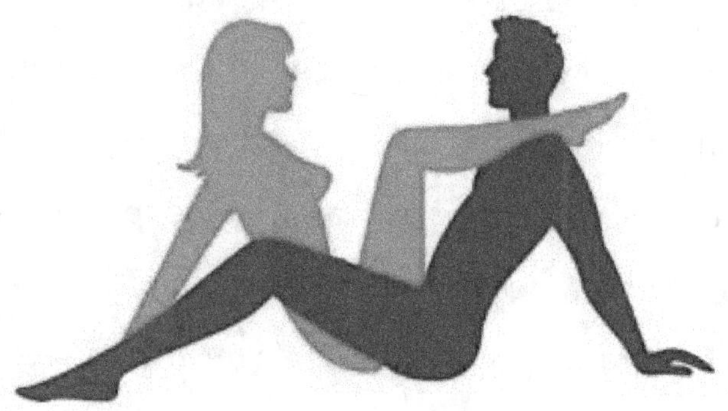

This is a position that requires patience and practice; however, it is rewarding once you get used to it. The lotus involves one partner (usually male) seated on a firm but soft surface, such as a bed or soft rug, with his legs folded (or cross-legged). As he becomes erect, his partner (usually female) will slowly descend onto him, with both feet placed firmly next to him so she can softly land onto him as he slips inside.

Once both are fully settled into this position, the woman's arms and legs are wrapped around the man, and he reciprocates with a similar embrace. This is a deeply intimate pose. The couple can look into each other's eyes at close proximity and embrace during the full experience of lovemaking. The woman can slightly lift and adjust within the position to gain a slightly different angle, which can allow her to experience more pleasure and possibly orgasm. To make this a successful pose, use a lot of lubrication and take it slow. This is not a position that accommodates a quick motion or thrust but rather a slower, more tantric pace.

The Butterfly

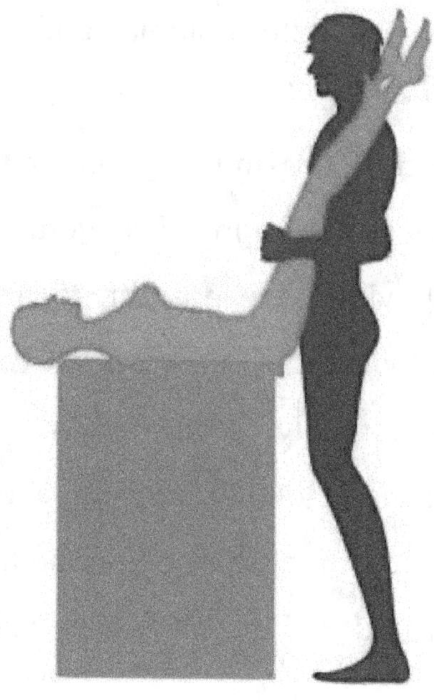

This position is a fun and ambitious pose that requires a bit of flexibility. In this pose, the man is standing, while the woman is lying on her back with her legs held in the air, though not too far apart, so as to be able to place each one on her partner's shoulders. In doing this, the man can easily penetrate and gently push against his partner's legs as he enters deeper.

This position gives the man a full view of the woman as he penetrates her; he can be standing at the edge of the bed during this process or with legs bent on the bed in the same fashion. For some women, keeping their legs slightly bent makes the transition into this position easier until they become more comfortable.

Three-Legged Dog

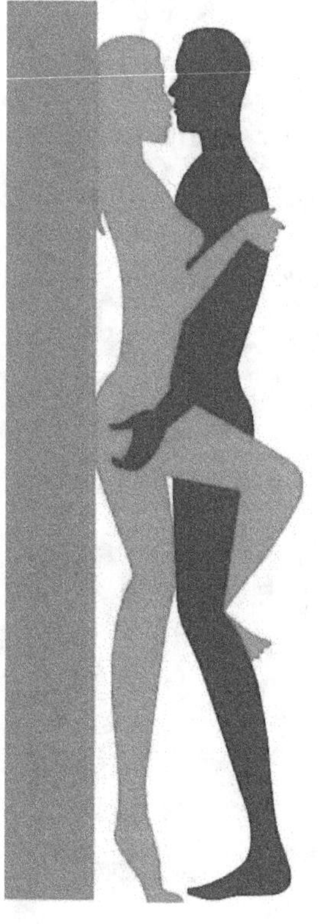

This position is done standing up, usually with one partner against a wall for added support, and one leg raised so that the partner can easily enter and penetrate. It is not the easiest feat to pull off, though it is fun despite the challenge, and can be done in a variety of places. For the woman, having her back against the wall is a good support during this pose.

Moreover, lifting one leg can be done with some support; the man holds and positions the lifted leg slightly higher or to the side so that he can enter easily. There is a bit of fine-tuning that involves figuring out at which angle is best to enter. Another variable to consider is the height of both individuals. If one person is taller (the male), it may be easier to enter when the woman is standing on a support or at a higher level. Alternatively, the male can bend or maneuver his position to lower his stance and accommodate a different height. This three-legged dog works easiest for people who are similar in height, though it can be achievable for anyone if you are willing to get creative and flexible (Emery, 2018).

The Hot Seat

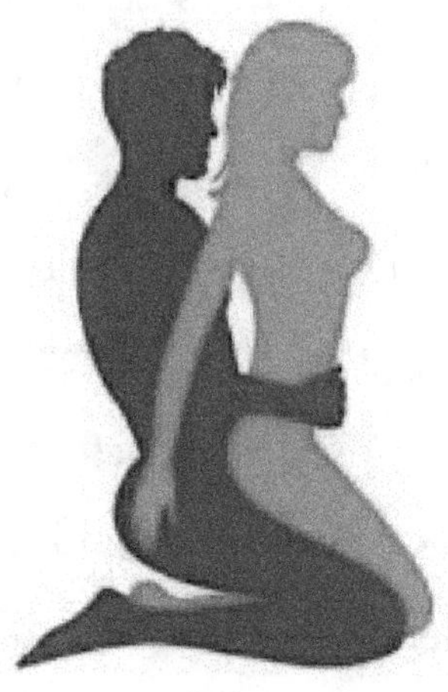

This position involves the man sitting in a kneeling position with his upper body leaning back, allowing for his partner, facing in the same direction and knelt in the same fashion, to slip her legs in between his, which are apart enough to enter inside from behind. As she leans back, they become closer, with his arms wrapping around her torso as she reaches for his waist from behind. This position works well in slow, steady motion.

Shameless

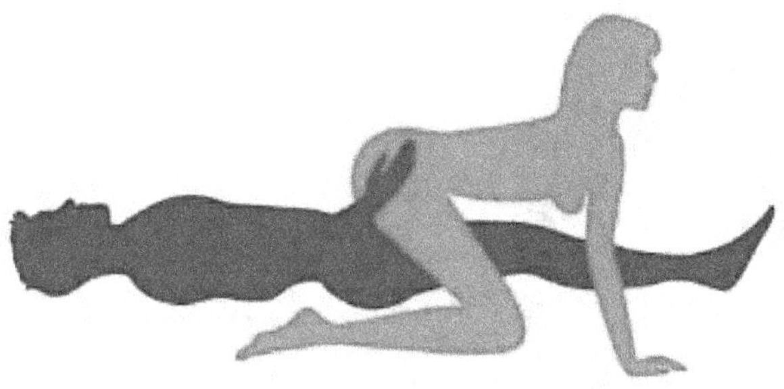

The man lies on his back, his legs are straight but slightly apart with his penis. The woman sits atop back to her lover. She leans forward and pins the lover to the bed and then begins moving back and forth, front to back.

Tantric Sex

What is tantric sex, and how can it improve lovemaking? Tantric sex originated from the tantric practice in Tibetan Buddhism, which began in India. It involves mediation and strengthening one's spirituality. The practice of tantric sex is closely associated with the pattern of mediation and connectivity. It incorporates sexual intimacy to create and enhance a deeper bond and experience with your partner. It is not a casual posture or technique. It requires study, meditation, and practice to achieve the best outcome and benefits.

The idea behind Tantra is to view every activity in life (such as eating, sex, or exercise) as a potential way to better oneself through self-realization and self-improvement. This applies similarly to mindful eating, where the practice of enjoying a meal is approached at a slower pace, taking the time to focus on the meal itself to avoid being distracted and rushing to finish. For exercise, there are various forms of yoga that apply to this practice.

The general idea is to enhance our natural energy and get the most out of it, resulting in a position experience. When this practice is applied to sexual intimacy, it can be a powerful and emotionally wonderful experience (Scaccia, 2018).

What are the common techniques in tantric sex? The idea of incorporating meditation and mindfulness during sex may seem like an unusual concept for some people, and while it does take a while to get used to, there are some important factors to understand before you begin:

1. *Slow down.* This practice is not for a quick session or fast-paced sexual activity. Reserve your tantric experience for when you have adequate time to explore and enjoy at a slow, comfortable pace.

2. *Practice.* Make sure you practice with your partner after you both have discussed it and agree fully to make it a goal. If only one person is in favor of this practice, it will not provide the full benefit for the couple as a whole.

3. *Try yoga and meditation.* Be familiar with the practice of slowing down and becoming mindful and aware of your surroundings, body, and mind. If you are new to these practices, it may be beneficial to join a class or try some beginner poses and movements with measured breathing techniques.

4. *Find a quiet, relaxing place.* Dim the lighting and add some candles. Essential oils, soft music, and any other instruments to help you unwind work well. You will want to experience a complete "letting go" of the mind and body while maintaining a mental focus on your partner. A gentle water fountain or the sounds of ocean water and birds can be ideal if you are outdoors, or simply find a sound clip and play it during your experience.

5. *Begin with meditation.* Try this before you engage with your partner to minimize any "noise" or distraction in your mind. During your meditation, take a body scan. Start with your head and note any tension or discomfort.

Release any tension in your body as you work your way down from your head through your jaws, neck, chest, and torso and continue until you reach your toes. Take your time and do not rush. By the time you reach your toes, your body should feel at ease, lighter than before, and ready for pleasure.

6. *Avoid any place with distractions and excessive noise.* You may find the comfort of a small urban space peaceful, as well as an outdoor space in a secluded beach or the woods. If you can't get far away, make use of your regular space. Minimize noise as much as possible, and allow yourself to focus on you and your partner.

In general, a tantric experience should feel as though all your stress melts away and arousal takes over with relaxation. It may take time to adjust to this form of lovemaking, as many people are used to more traditional and possibly quicker ways of getting intimate. Beginners to tantric sex should try scheduling one session alone with their partner weekly, even if it is just for one or two hours.

If your life is busy, find an open space in the evening or during the weekend, when life slows down a bit and allows you to enjoy a more relaxed pace for a while (Surnow, 2016).

How to Practice Tantric Sex

It is not as complicated or mysterious as you may think, and it takes more time and patience to achieve the desired results once you decide to give it a try. When you begin, take your time to watch cues from your partner and how they respond. Any hesitation or uncertainty should be responded to with care and consideration. Let your partner know that you are aiming to please them and to make the experience enjoyable for both.

1. Breathe slowly and evenly. Allow yourself to draw your breath in, counting to five, then exhale at the same slow and measured breath.

2. Move slowly and gently. Think of slowing down and gradually getting into the groove with movement. Set a pace that takes a quick thrust or

action, and move in a deeper, slower motion than you may be used to.

3. Make sure you and your partner are both comfortable and relaxed before proceeding. If there are any doubts or uncertainties, these should be discussed openly before any tantric activities.

4. Use touch and gentle communication to practice new poses and motions. Don't rush into any positions that seem challenging at first. Start with something simple and work your way into more intricate poses.

Tantric Sex: What It Is and Isn't

There are some common misconceptions about tantric sex and how it works. It may seem like a new but strange approach to sex for some people and a welcome change for others who are looking to enhance the romantic side of their life.

Tantric sex can take on various forms and patterns, depending on how you and your partner choose to enjoy it. For example, some couples will read books on many poses and movements and try each one, while others will stick with a few simple positions at first to try it out and become comfortable before proceeding further.

What tantric sex is not:

1. It is not a fad, despite many people feeling this way because of its notoriety among celebrities and as a result of its surge in popularity. Tantric sex and meditation techniques date back thousands of years, and while it may seem new and "in" now, it has been practiced for centuries, at least variations of it.

2. It is not expensive. You do not have to make any investments in pricy books, props, background music, or natural diffusers to achieve what tantric sex is meant to do for you and your partner.

3. It is not a marathon of sorts that requires you or your partner to try every position and technique within the practice. The choice is completely open and can be modified according to your ability and preference. For example, some poses are difficult to achieve for some people who suffer from chronic pain or injuries that make certain motions or poses painful and difficult.

What tantric sex is:

1. It is fun, peaceful, and relaxing. It increases the level of connection and intimacy with your partner.

2. It is an effective way to achieve a deeper level of intimacy while reducing stress and blood pressure. There are numerous benefits to a regular exercise routine, and tantric sex can become a central role in this.

3. It is a way to achieve a strong level of mindfulness and peace through intimacy. Sex plays an important role in a relationship. In the next chapters, you will learn the many

techniques to make sex an amazing experience beyond the ordinary routine that many people get stuck in. Taking the time and effort to try new and exciting ideas in the context of lovemaking is an ideal way to bond well with your partner and make your sex life the best it can be!

Chapter 5: The Warm-Up

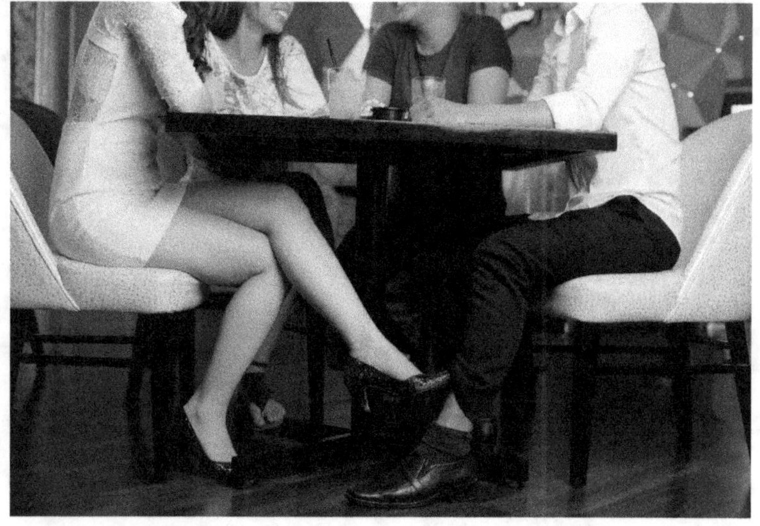

Foreplay is an important part of getting "warmed up" for a good session with your partner. Getting in the mood does not happen automatically for everyone, and jumping into the act of sex is not the best method for most people who need a chance to get acquainted with their sensual side first. Kissing, touching, and holding your partner are common ways to get closer to them. Show them your interest in taking things further. There are also specific ways to get better acquainted with your body and your partner's during foreplay. This involves learning about the erogenous zones. These are the areas of your body that provide a tingling sensation or heightened sense of arousal, more so than other parts of your body. Some of these areas may not be as obvious as you may think, which makes them more important to learn about and practice touching and playing with.

How do you know if your partner is in the mood, and how can you guide them with seduction? For new lovers or partners, seduction is relatively easy because you are in a new and exciting relationship full of arousal and intimacy.

For couples who have been together for a while, there are challenges of routine and becoming so involved in life's business that getting down to business can be less frequent and without the same level of thrill and spontaneity that used to be a part of your lovemaking. There are some easy and fun ways to get the fire going, and these ways can also be applied to newer couples looking to try new ways of seduction to get their partner's attention.

1. *Tease your partner.* Make them curious about what you have in mind. They may respond in kind, teasing you as well, and this will mount to seduction, eventually foreplay and further action.

2. *Make a move.* It could even be a slight one when it is least expected. This could be a bold move but also one that gets your partner's attention. This could mean a teasing brush of the hand in an erogenous area of your partner's body at a public event, discreetly, or while you are both watching a movie and beginning to relax. The unexpected aspect of this move is what makes it exciting, as it takes you by surprise.

The element of surprise is a strong motivation to go with a new and exciting adventure.

3. *Surprise your partner.* You can prepare a special dinner at home by candlelight or plan a weekend away, just the two of you. If you are not used to taking the initiative, this is a good way to start and give your partner a pleasant surprise when they least expect it.

4. *Plan a fun role-playing event with your partner.* This can be organized in conjunction with a weekend getaway or an evening away from home. One example of how this can be arranged is pretending to be strangers in a pub and meeting for the first time. You may play different roles and have a hot night of passion afterward. This may seem unusual or strange to imagine, especially if you have never attempted role-playing. However, with a new (or different) set of clothes, scene, and a sense of imagination, this experience can be memorable and exciting at once.

5. *Switch roles.* If your partner is often the one who takes charge in the relationship, offer to be the one who takes the initiative.

Alternatively, if you are the one to initiate and direct the show, give the power to your partner for the night and see what happens (Marin, 2016).

Finding Your Erogenous Zones

There are specific erogenous zones that your partner and you can experiment with for sensation and touch. These areas of the body contain a high concentration of nerves that make them highly sensitive so that even the slightest graze of a finger or tip of the tongue on your skin will create a tingling sensation throughout your body. For this reason, it is important to identify these regions of the body to enhance pleasure during foreplay and sex. At first glance, many people may skip these areas of the body as they are not considered sexual or associated with sex initially. It is important to realize that sensuality and the subtlety of light touching and tracing can have a powerful effect on the body's response system. It can result in immediate arousal with just a slight touch or movement within seconds.

It is a quick way to turn someone on, and while some people are more sensitive to touch than others, most people will respond favorably to being caressed or traced lightly in the erogenous areas of the body (Krisher, n.d.).

Erogenous Zones in Men

There are erogenous zones specifically important in men. Some of these regions are obvious, while others may seem unlikely or lesser-known. Once you know which areas of the body help your partner respond well, you will greatly improve the foreplay experience.

1. The penis. The first and most obvious area considered an erogenous zone for men is the penis. It has a lot of nerves that heighten sensitivity, making the slightest brush or touch to cause an immediate response. Caressing the penis is an easy way to get things started, and it gives your partner the direct approach of saying, "I'm interested right now."

2. *The nape of the neck.* This region is also sensitive to the slightest touch, and it can create a quick response, signaling interest in exploring more.

During foreplay, this part of the body is an excellent start. You can also begin with the sides of the neck or cheek, lightly kissing your partner and working from there. The trail of kisses, once extended to the neck, becomes more intense as you reach the nape.

Your partner will reciprocate in the same way, as this zone is very sensual for women as well.

3. *The scalp.* This is a tender and responsive area, whether you give your partner a scalp massage with your fingertips or smooth their hair with your hands. It can be a desirable part of the body to enjoy during foreplay.

4. *The nipples.* These are not only sensitive for women but men too. Once men notice this, they may enjoy a light nipple massage or licking in the general area. This is a great way to get the arousal growing, which can lead to more kissing and/or a trail of kisses down below for some oral fun.

Erogenous Zones in Women

Women share some of the same erogenous zones as men, which makes it easier for both partners to identify them on each other. If it pleases him, it may have the same effect on the woman as well.

1. The vagina. There is a G-spot inside the vagina, which is clustered with nerve endings. Deep penetration is a way to stimulate this area to achieve a satisfying orgasm.

While it is not going to be part of the initial foreplay stages, it can be a goal during the sexual experience.

2. The clitoris. One of the most sensitive and pleasurable parts of a woman's body, the clitoris can create a sexual response, including a full orgasm. Licking, touching, or kissing this part of the body and the region directly around it is a sure way to get your partner interested.

3. *The inner side of the wrist.* This is an area with a lot of nerve endings, making it a tender spot to touch and tease. Even an accidental brush on the wrist can conjure up some arousal for a woman and cause a receptive response right away. It can be subtle but effective at the same time.

4. *The nape of the neck.* Similar to men, this part is another strong erogenous zone for women. In fact, a couple can easily become aroused with neck play alone, combined with kissing and petting.

5. *The inner thighs.* These are tender areas that can arouse a woman with a gentle brush of the finger or hand. This is a great way to initiate oral sex or manual stimulation during foreplay.

Both men and women share a lot of the same erogenous areas, which makes foreplay and arousal easy to coordinate and enjoy for both. Some people may become ticklish or feel more or less sensation in certain zones than others.

For many people, the erogenous zones are revisited and cherished throughout the lovemaking process. The heightened level of sensitivity can work wonders during sex and make your experience more worthwhile as a result.

Chapter 6: Masturbation

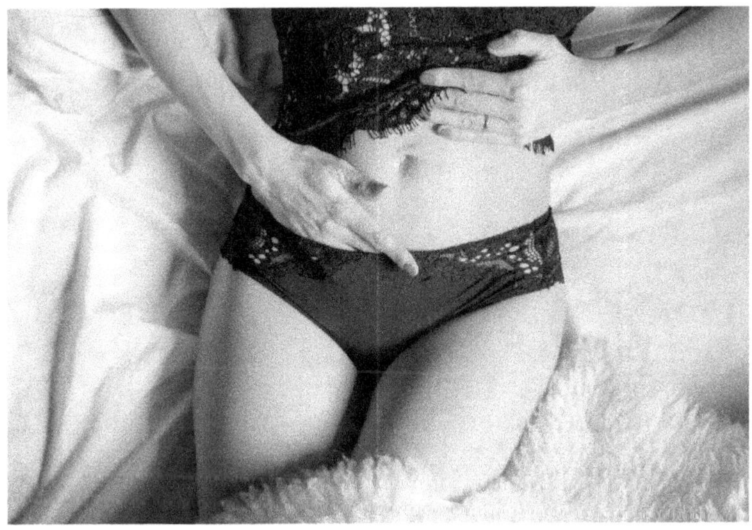

Pleasuring yourself is an important part of learning about what brings pleasure to you sexually. It is an opportunity to explore your body and the sensations you experience through various forms of touch, such as caressing and tickling. Masturbation can be enjoyed solo or with your partner. There are several ways to approach self-pleasuring as a couple. You can manually stimulate each other or observe your partner play as you do the same. It is an important way of showing your partner exactly where and how you like to be stimulated.

Masturbation with Your Partner

Mutual masturbation is self-pleasuring together with your partner. It can be done either individually with yourself next to your partner as they do the same or masturbating each other by touching and caressing each other's genitals during the process. This is a great opportunity for both partners to get acquainted with each other's bodies and to learn what makes them excited.

Observing your partner masturbate gives you a lesson on where they like to be stimulated and how they enjoy being touched. They may invite you to pleasure them, too, or simply ask you to watch, which can prompt you to do the same. There are some important and interesting facts to consider before mutual masturbation with your partner:

1. It is safe and fun, and the boundaries are clear for both. Some people are more autoerotic by nature, which means they enjoy playing with themselves and giving pleasure to their bodies instead of having someone else do this.

2. You can use toys, props, and lubricants to customize your fun. With your partner nearby, you can both enjoy trying new techniques and sensations. This not only allows you to observe each other but ourselves as well.

3. It is a great option when penetration is not an option or preference.

4. There are fewer risks of STIs (sexually transmitted infections).

Getting acquainted with mutual masturbation is a great alternative to other forms of sex. It can involve a lot of toys and options or just your partner and you. It can fit well into life in between other forms of sex or in place of them.

Self-Pleasuring While Solo (Men)

Masturbation is a common way for men to enjoy pleasure solo, and they often do so quickly when they find a discrete spot, whether it is at home, work, or somewhere they can easily get off without any interruption. The biological nature of men makes masturbation more accessible than for women, who need a bit more room or creativity to maneuver around small spaces. While self-pleasuring is often manual, using one or both hands, there are some ideas to consider for playing:

1. Lotions and lubricants definitely enhance the experience for men. There is a variety of lubes available, from cooling sensations to warming.

2. Cock rings are useful for helping an erection last longer than usual. Some men use specifically shaped rings to stimulate the perineum during play.

3. Prostate stimulation can be done with the use of stimulator or plug, which can provide an added benefit while masturbating at the same time.

4. Manually stroking and fondling the penis and testicles is the most common method of self-play. Electronic and manual toys to stimulate the prostate and/or perineum are both great options for enhancing the experience (James, n.d.).

Self-Pleasuring While Solo (Women)

Women often masturbate and enjoy it just as much as men. The challenges for women are the positioning and space needed to adequately self-pleasure and get the most out of their bodies. A comfortable space is best, which is both quiet and easy to relax.

Masturbating in a small space can present a hurdle, though it can be managed with some creativity. One of the most central features of masturbation is the clitoris. It has a number of nerve endings that create a tingling sensation when stimulated. During self-pleasuring, this area is generally the most enjoyable, though there are a number of surrounding areas that can be teased, stroked, and brushed for arousal to get things started.

1. Play with your clitoris and labia with soft strokes of the fingers, gradually spreading and exploring in between with circular motions and strokes.

2. The motion of your hand and fingers can vary to achieve the desired effect. It can be from side to side or up and down. Work with the motion that gives you the most pleasure.

3. Use lube and apply to the labia to achieve a smooth, slippery feel, and stroke it more to get a warm feeling. Try various motions, and you will gradually find yourself developing stronger arousal and wetness.

4. Squeeze, pinch, and tickle yourself. Trace your fingers from your inner thigh into your labia, and treat yourself to some anticipation with your own touch.

There are some props you might want to introduce into your self-play routine:

1. A shower head can be an intense and enjoyable way to enhance stimulation, either as part of your shower or in the bathtub.

2. A dildo or sex toy can be used to rub against the clitoris and labia, as well as penetration. Make sure you use a lot of lubrication to make the experience more enjoyable.

3. A long string of pearls or similar jewelry can be used to rub against your body. If another piece of jewelry is used instead of pearls, be sure to choose something that doesn't have any clasps or sharp chains that can cause scraping and discomfort (Jameson, n.d.).

Chapter 7: Oral Sex

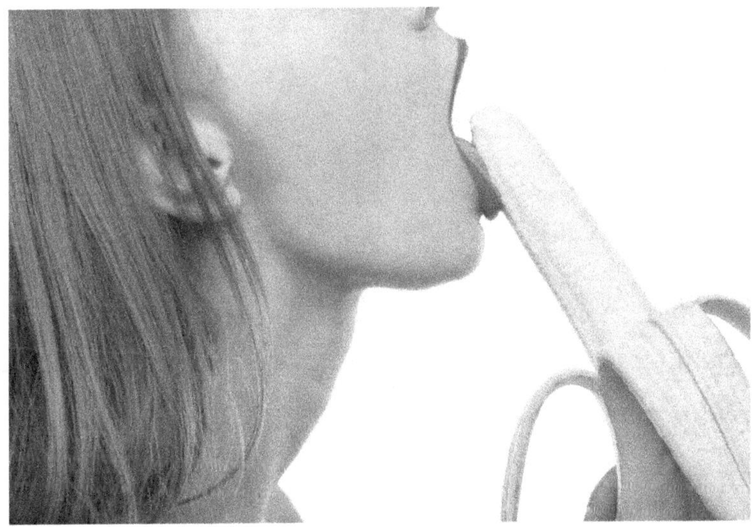

Oral sex is a personal and enjoyable experience between partners that can bring about a powerful orgasm and an enjoyable sense of connection. For women, most orgasms do not occur during vaginal sex, and oral stimulation is one of the most important ways to achieve this result. Oral sex is one of the most pleasurable aspects of sex for many people, and learning new and interesting techniques will create more dimension to your sex life and experiences.

Tips for Oral Sex

Whether it is a blowjob or cunnilingus, oral sex is amazing in giving your partner a dose of individual attention to their needs and helping them achieve climax along the way. Oral stimulation does this on a sensitive level: one partner experiences the taste of their lover while pleasing them with their tongue and mouth. There are some important points to keep in mind before you begin.

1. Listen to your partner. They may or may not be ready when you are, and if they are, listen to what they say and look for cues. A stroke of the tongue in one area of the genitals can be pleasurable for some and annoying or uneventful for someone else. The best method? Ask your partner what they like.

2. Make long strokes with your tongue. Do so slowly so that your partner feels the full experience of you tasting them.

3. Vocalize. Encourage your partner to talk dirty during sex, or just let them describe or vocalize how they feel during the process. Let them direct you how to pleasure them, and ask them how, when, and to what degree. A light stroke in one area that may be sensitive can easily turn into a nibble or stronger thrust of the tongue because of the level of sensitivity.

4. It is not all tongue action! Use your fingers and nose to caress, and take mini breaks to check in but jump right back into action to keep your partner satisfied.

5. Don't stop! Keep the momentum going, and make sure your partner is responding with positive cues.

If at any point, there are any changes in their reaction or they want you to stop, do so immediately and ask what they like and do not like.

Techniques for Her Pleasure

Bringing your partner to orgasm is a wonderful experience that both lovers can enjoy together. The woman will relish the climax and the methods used to bring her to that state. Finding the right techniques can be a challenge for some people who lack experience. Thus, it is important to listen to your partner and ensure she gets the most out of it. The following tips are ideas that will help get your woman in a good position for enjoying oral pleasure:

1. Vary your tongue movements. Stimulate the labia and clitoris, making sure to cover the entire area. Note your partner's reaction to certain spots. If one specific area produces a moan or favorable response, continue with this technique. Alternatively, if one or more areas are uncomfortable or irritate your lover, avoid them. Stop briefly to ask if it is acceptable to continue, and ask for simple guidance on where to continue.

2. *Avoid stopping unless you or your partner need to adjust your position.* Most women enjoy lying on their backs with their legs apart, though there are some other positions that work well, such as squatting over their partner or standing up. Keep the momentum going with regular attention, and don't forget to check in briefly to make sure she's getting aroused.

3. *Try a variety of positions and settings.* Oral sex may be fun in bed, but it can be just as fun or more so in the shower, on a sofa, on a table or chair, or on other furniture. Always make sure your partner is comfortable and relaxed during the process so that arousal comes easily.

4. *Use a variety of techniques with your tongue and fingers.* Move around and try new motions, strokes, and circular moves. Avoid repeating the same motion over and over again, especially if your partner is not responsive to it or seems not to favor it.

5. *Anal and/or vaginal play can be incorporated during cunnilingus with the use of sex toys.* A simple vibrator or dildo can be one option. You may also use a butt plug.

Be sure to add a good amount of lubrication and give your partner a chance to adjust their position before inserting a toy. Take cues from your partner if they enjoy this additional play or if they want to change how it is done. After a few sessions, you will both get accustomed to what works and how to approach further pleasure in the future.

Techniques for His Pleasure

Like pleasuring a woman, you should always take cues from him and find out what makes him excited and aroused. For some men, they enjoy a lot of tongue action and stroking, while others want a deeper action, entering more orally and feeling a sense of suction or being engulfed, like during vaginal sex. A variance or shift between several methods can help gauge how well your partner receives each technique. The following tips are important to keep in mind and add to your experience:

1. Make eye contact with him and let him know you want to please. This does not have to be continuous, but looking up every now and then will reassure him that you are there to give him the best, plus it shows that you are watching his reaction, which gives him the opportunity to indicate or direct how to pleasure him with specific moves.

2. Take it slow, and speed up only when the moment is right. If your partner is growing closer to climax, it helps to move more vigorously and use a tighter grip, either with your mouth or with the assistance of your hands.

3. Vary the movements with your tongue. You may spell words or trace shapes to keep it interesting. Repeating the same motions can become monotonous, and any sign of arousal can drop significantly when this happens. Keep it fresh and interesting, and your partner will thank you for it.

4. If your partner is open to trying anal play, insert a finger to gauge his comfort level. Use lubrication to ensure there is no skin irritation and move slowly, either inserting or sliding in and out gently or more vigorously. Using different toys, either manual or electronic, can really increase the sensation, especially coupled with oral sex.

5. Take cues from your partner about what turns him on and what doesn't. Do not be afraid to ask or motion to try something new. Some techniques will work better than others.

Enjoying Oral Pleasure Together as a Couple

Enjoying the pleasure of oral sex together as a couple can be an excellent way to get better acquainted with each other's bodies and what turns you on. It also gives both lovers a chance to experience climax together, which is more likely done by simultaneously pleasuring each other than with vaginal sex. One of the most popular positions used by couples is the 69, where one partner lies on their back and the other lies over them, in reverse, giving both lovers access to each other for oral pleasure. When you are new to trying this method, there are a few new discoveries you may encounter:

1. One partner can easily get distracted by their own arousal and slow down from pleasuring the other. This can be easily remedied by continuing again. This normally happens with most people. Over time, it gets easier to multitask giving while receiving.

2. Use both hands and your mouth to pleasure your partner. A 69 position gives both partners opportunities to move their bodies to adjust according to which methods work. For example, if you are typically on top, you will have more use of your upper body, arms, and hands. On the bottom, you can slip your arms over or through one or both legs of your partner to play and experiment.

3. Stay consistent with each other so that you can bring yourselves to orgasm relatively within the same time span. This is not always easily achieved, but it is one of the best experiences you will have once you do! This requires a close amount of contact and using cues and communication to let your partner know where you are in the process. This will give them an idea of how close you are to climax and how close or far they are in comparison.

4. Add some anal play while giving and receiving pleasure. This is something that can be used to heighten an already highly charged state of arousal. If anal play is new to one or both lovers, start off slow.

Discuss the possibilities in advance so that there are no surprises or disagreements during the session, which can ruin the fun altogether.

Where can you both give and receive oral sex? The bedroom is the first option for many who find the flat surface of the bed easy to move and position the body for maximum comfort. For more adventure, try the sofa, floor, or shower. More flexible and athletic couples may try a handstand or dangle off a structure (make sure it is a stable, permanent fixture!) while being pleasured and providing oral sex at the same time. Mutual masturbation can often lead to oral sex with one partner satisfying the other manually while the other does the same orally until one reaches orgasm. There is the option of switching back and forth to get the best of both types of stimulation.

There are some variations of the 69 position that can enhance your experience. You can engage on your sides with your legs opened in a scissor fashion. If one partner is typically on top, it can be fun to switch positions partway through each session.

You will find that some variations work better than others, and one may be more favorable to one partner than the other. While it is good to try to work through many options to explore, you will eventually settle on one or two favorite positions (Manley, 2019).

Fisting for Pleasure: The Undiscovered Joy

Most people cringe or avoid the idea of fisting, as it seems to cause pain and discomfort and unlikely to arouse. In reality, most people who do try it may be hasty and unprepared. That is one reason why it is avoided, just like anal sex, which is covered in chapter 11. Why is fisting enjoyable and what aspect of it makes people intrigued? Having a large fist inside provides the feeling of fullness and stimulates a lot of nerves and tissues on a deeper level. It is a practice that should be done slowly and with a lot of lubrication, as it is an intense and full experience.

Vaginal fisting can be enjoyable and arousing beyond your expectations, and the person using the fist should also feel comfortable and relaxed doing so, as this is a process that should be done slowly.

The following are tips for fisting and getting the most out of it:

1. *Make sure you have more than enough lube.* You might want to have more than double the amount: think of two tubes. It doesn't hurt to be prepared and ready to be generous with it. Adding more is better than having less and causing irritation and chafing

2. *Use latex gloves with the lube.* Have fun with different colors and styles, and try different scenarios, such as role-playing a medical exam, as some people may enjoy them in certain situations.

3. *Try different shapes with the fingers.* The first shape and easiest to accept is where all fingers are pressed together, forming a "beak" shape with your hand. This will give your partner a chance to gradually accept and expand to engulf the fist or hand completely.

4. *Take it slow and watch your partner's reaction.* Are they enjoying the experience, or is it too much? If at any time, the experience becomes painful or difficult for your partner, assure them you will stop, then do so by pulling out slowly and carefully. Not everyone will get a thrill from this activity, even if they are eager to give it a try!

5. *Finally, discuss this activity in advance.* Make sure you are both interested in the same way without any coercing or pushing. This is a deeply satisfying experience for some, but not everyone will be on board. For this reason, take the time to get familiar with your partner's interests and needs first, which may or may not include fisting (Thomas, 2017).

Chapter 8: Best Positions for Female Orgasm

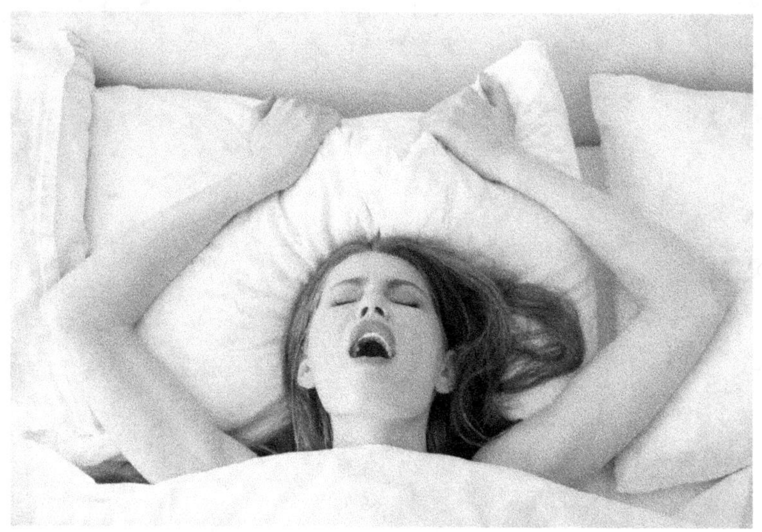

To achieve an orgasm, determining your position and how you wish to enjoy reaching a climax is important. Typically, women reach orgasm by oral sex or cunnilingus or manually through stimulation by themselves or with their partner. During vaginal sex, there is a G-spot that can be accessed through deep penetration, which is achievable with several positions.

The amount of stimulation of the clitoris and foreplay also play a major role in how successful orgasm is to achieve. Achieving orgasm can be done by covering your bases as follows:

1. *Clitoral stimulation.* Stimulate the clitoris as much as possible before and during sex. This will keep the area engorged, full of blood, and highly sensitive throughout the session.

While clitoral play is excellent during foreplay, it works even better during vaginal sex. Some women find that stimulating the clitoris prior to sex is a good way to achieve orgasm later during vaginal sex.

Try any position that allows for the penis to rub or brush against the clitoris during vaginal penetration to achieve orgasm at the same time. This can be challenging, though achievable, for some couples.

2. *Deep penetration of the penis.* This will bring about orgasm by reaching the g-spot inside, which is full of nerve endings. This is done by having sex in a doggy-style position, which allows for deeper entrance and penetration. It allows the woman more movement, giving her the option of pushing back against her partner and adjusting her legs closer or further apart, to make the most of the experience.

3. *Woman on top.* When the woman is on top, she has the ability to shift her body and gliding angle to reach further and deeper. This gives her the control, but also the freedom to shift according to how she experiences stimulation.

4. *Varied poses.* Couples can use a variety of side poses, where the man enters the woman from behind, and allows for a range of motion to shift around for deeper penetration.

The woman is also free to stimulate the clitoris during vaginal sex, giving her more opportunity to reach orgasm.

What is the best way to achieve orgasm for women? Is it through vaginal, oral, or other forms of sex? The key is to communicate and learn what works and what doesn't. If one method seems to progress toward orgasm faster, keep this in mind. Using lubrication is always a good idea, especially if you plan on trying or switching between various positions during one session.

This can be hard on the skin, and a little warmth and lubrication can go a long way to avoid a lot of discomforts. Do not be afraid to try different methods and explore new possibilities with your partner, even if they seem unlikely, as they could open a new door to trying a variety of new techniques and sensations.

Finally, it is normal not to achieve orgasm sometimes. This can be for a variety of reasons and not just physical but psychological as well.

Therefore, it is important to be patient and take your time with your partner so that you can both get the most out of the experience (Klepchukova, 2019).

Positions

The Hero:

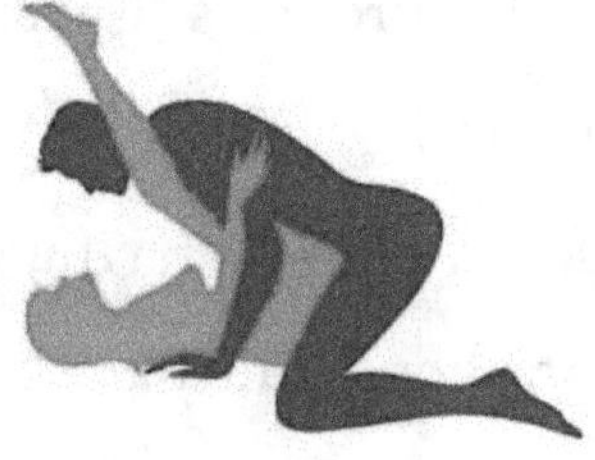

Suspended congress:

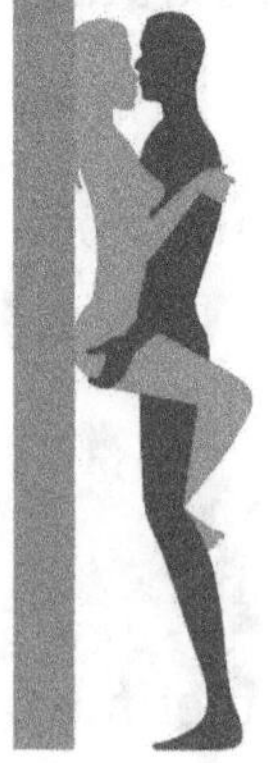

The Queen:

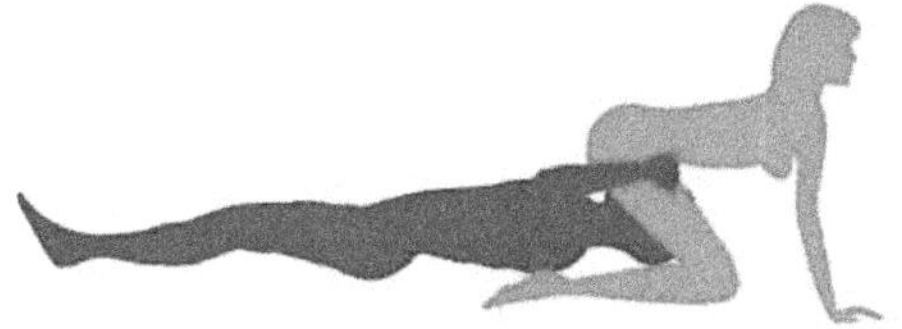

Leg Gilder:

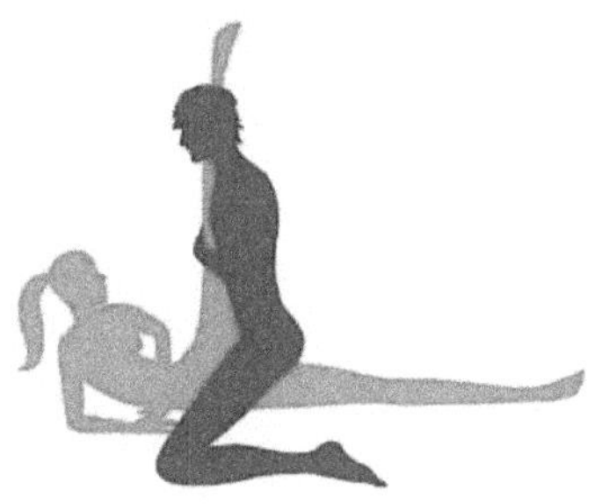

Victory:

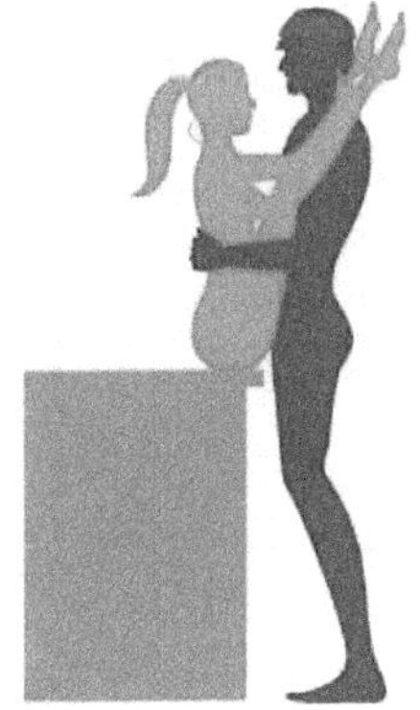

Chapter 9: Best Positions for Male Orgasm

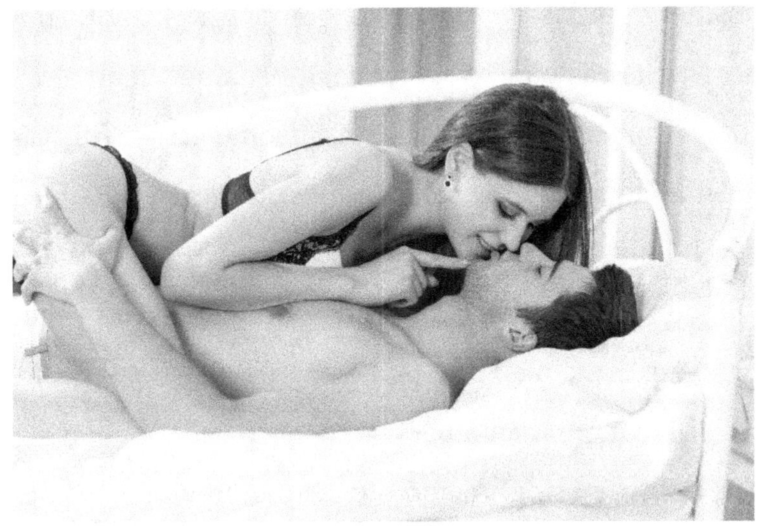

Men often have more options when it comes to finding the right position for orgasm. It may actually seem like men can climax anywhere and everywhere, given their biology and ease at which they can pleasure themselves. Vaginal sex and anal sex give men the advantage when they penetrate as they are fully engaged and can experience this in many different positions and scenarios. It is important to note that despite its easy and opportune appearance, many men struggle with reaching orgasm in some cases. This can be due to many reasons, some physical and others psychological. Some men can experience orgasm without ejaculation through stimulation of their prostate. Some men find that certain scenarios or events stimulate more than others.

The following tips are good to keep in mind for helping him achieve the best orgasm possible:

1. *Giving a handjob.* Start with a handjob before oral or other forms of sex. This will give him an advantage before starting. He may want to participate or let you take control.

2. *Slowing down.* During the course of sex, if he is getting close to ejaculating but wants to prolong the climax to enjoy it more, slow down the pace. This can slow down his progression as well and make it easier for him to gain more control over ejaculation and when to climax. This can allow for more pleasure leading up to the orgasm.

3. *Communicating.* Open dialogue and discussion about how to move or position with your partner can make a big difference in the level of enjoyment. He may already know how to make the most out of his climax, or he may want to explore a few different methods first.

4. *Engaging the kegel muscles.* Your kegel muscles are helpful in massaging the penis vaginally during sex. Kegels are muscles that can be strengthened with regular exercise, and they make a significant impact during sex with him. He will notice a "milking" sensation, which gives him a deeper sensation of being gripped. This can help bring about a more intense orgasm. This practice can also be applied with anal sex, as this area tends to tighten more.

Discover new positions and methods of play to get the most out of orgasm, and make it worthwhile for him (Eliason, n.d.).

Positions

The Frog:

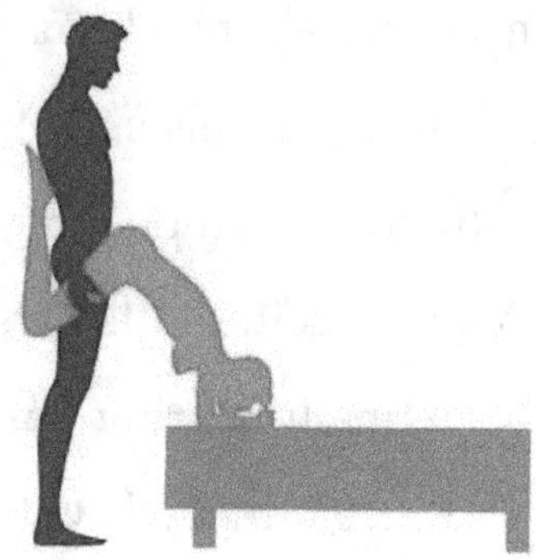

Jet Driver:

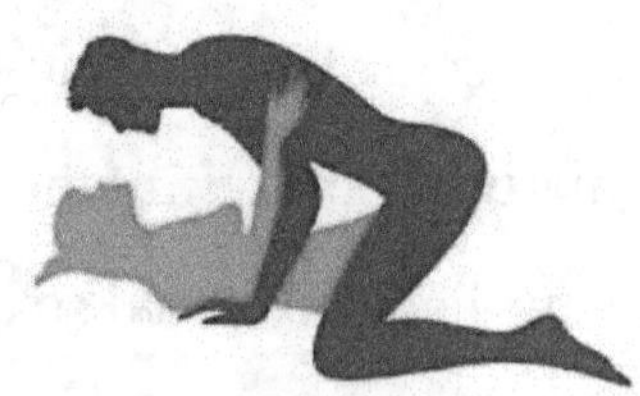

The Elevator:

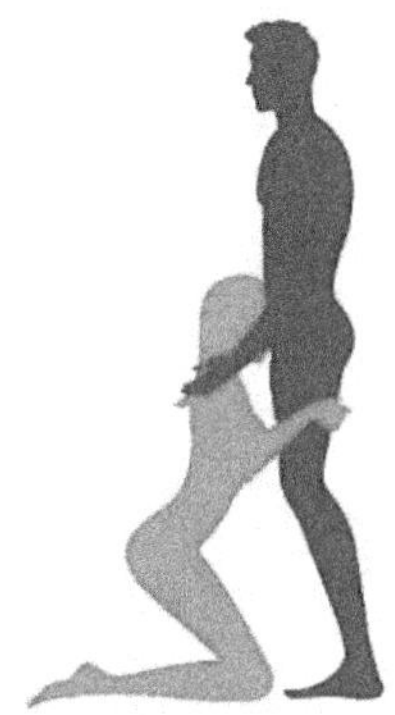

Rear Entry:

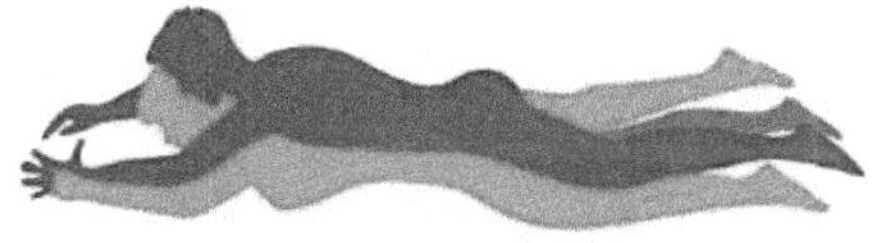

Straight Concubine:

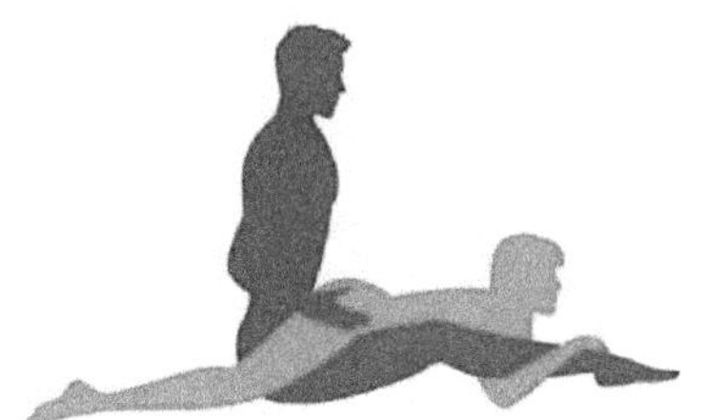

Close Binding

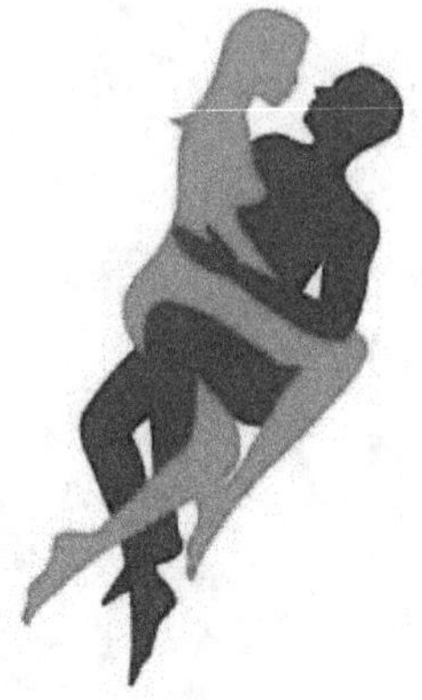

Chapter 10: Double Pleasure

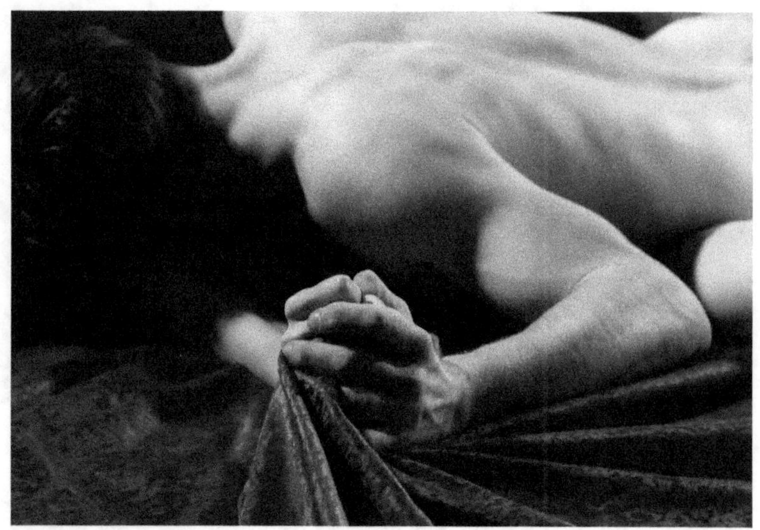

Experiencing orgasm simultaneously or together may seem like a dream or a fantasy come true! It may also seem unlikely and unrealistic, considering how men and women reach orgasm in different ways and not always in the same position and at the same time.

There are a number of positions that can bring a lot of pleasure to both lovers.

1. *Reverse cowgirl position.* This involves the woman mounting on top, with her back to her partner. This can be done by straddling one or both legs. This position allows the woman to have control over how she moves on top while the man has the benefit of lying back and enjoying the sensation.

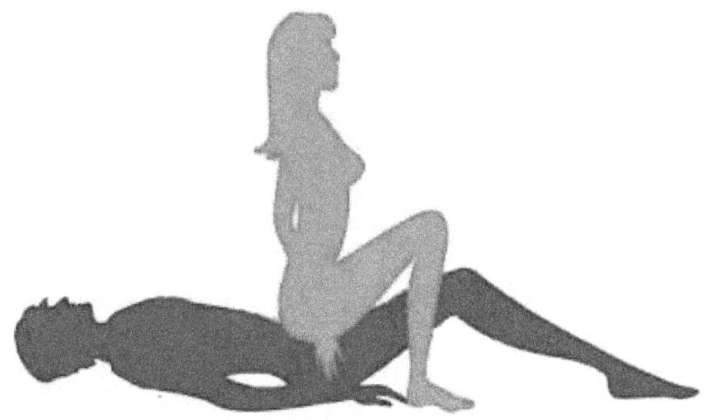

2. *Doggy style.* A variation on the doggy-style position is to use your elbows to prop your upper body as your partner enters from behind. This alters the position to where the woman can experience deeper penetration and achieve orgasm along with the man.

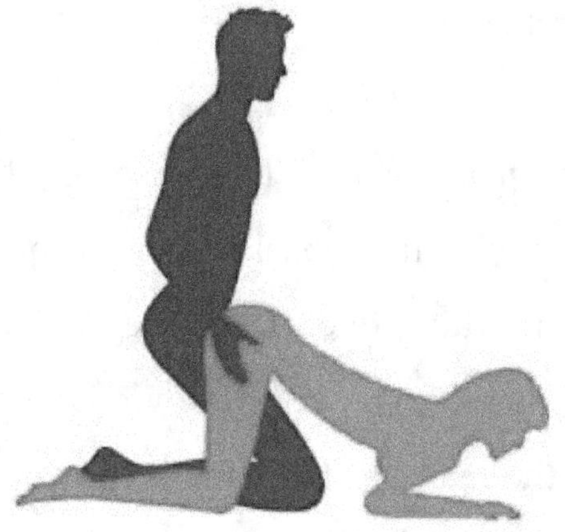

3. *Oral sex.* This is one of the best ways to achieve orgasm simultaneously, together with manual stimulation through mutual masturbation. This can be combined with many positions to heighten the arousal and bring about climax for both partners quickly.

Achieving Multiple Orgasms

Some couples are able to achieve multiple orgasms through a variety of different positions, including the options for double orgasms, where both partners experience climax together. For women, this is often done through oral or manual stimulation, while men tend to achieve this through vaginal or anal sex. The best way to practice multiple orgasms is to self-pleasure until this happens. It may take a while, and with the increase of intensity, some people may pull away to relish the experience. For others, continuing to play during the first orgasm will lead to more, one after the other.

Chapter 11: Anal Sex

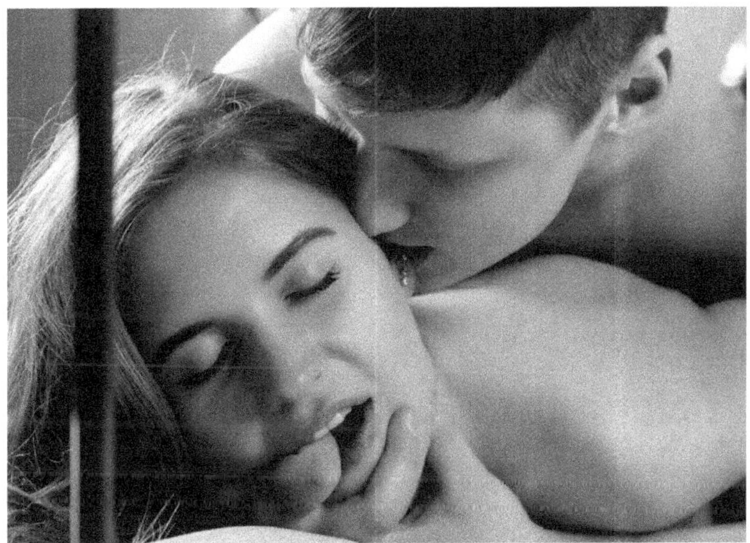

Anal sex is an activity that can be enjoyed by both men and women. Although it is often misunderstood and surrounded by myths and misperceptions, it can be an incredible sense of pleasure once you become comfortable with it. One of the most important aspects of anal sex is establishing a good comfort level with your partner. You should both be able to freely express any concerns or sensations during this practice but also before you start. Once you clear away any inhibitions about anal sex, you will be able to explore the amazing possibilities and enjoyment. It is not something to rush into but rather a practice that progresses slowly.

Helpful Tips for a Pleasurable Anal Sex

Helpful tips and suggestions to make anal sex easier to enjoy can involve a number of variations and movements so that everything fits just right. Below a few tips you will find helpful to make the process enjoyable:

1. Be honest. Honesty about your feelings and experience during all stages of anal sex is important. Tell your partner when it becomes too uncomfortable and when a break is needed. It can take time to become accustomed to it, and some people are more adaptable than others.

2. *Lubricate.* Before you begin, invest in good-quality lubrication. This is an absolute necessity to make the process easier and safer. Find a lubricant that works best for you and your partner, especially if allergies are an issue and/or sensitivity. Lubrication is a must and should always be used during all forms of sex. This is especially important for anal penetration, which should be done with patience and a great deal of care.

3. *Relax.* Make sure you and your partner feel relaxed. This process can take time to get used to, but once you do, it only gets better with time.

4. *Try a rim job.* This is basically providing oral sex to the anus opening. This can get your partner in the mood for anal play and can be done while the lube is ready to apply as well.

5. Use pillows, blankets, and other soft objects. Make your experience as comfortable as possible to avoid injury or rubbing from rough or difficult surfaces. Some bedding can seem soft but may chafe or scrape the skin hard after repetitive motion. Using a table or chair, for example, can be a challenge. Make sure that it has some soft cushioning to avoid rubbing against a hard or grainy surface (Jameson, n.d.).

Great Positions for Anal Sex

Anal sex can be an enjoyable part of your love life, and there are many positions that can add to the pleasure. Some require a bit more flexibility than others. However, with some practice, many of them can become part of your enjoyment.

1. The "jet driver" position. This involves the recipient lying on their back, lifting their back up and draping their legs over their head and shoulders. It gives their partner full control to insert and penetrate. However, it is a difficult position to hold unless you have a good balance. To make it easier, use pillows and blankets as props to keep in place.

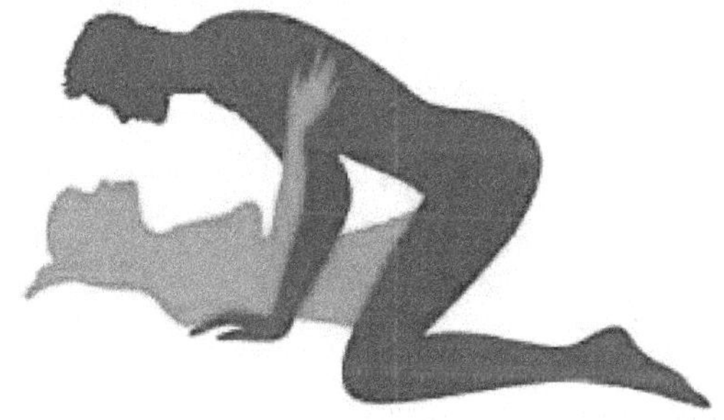

2. *The doggy-style position.* It is excellent, as it allows for some motion and variations to get comfortable and enjoy the sensation. A simpler and easier position to try first is a variation on the doggy-style position, in which one person lies on their tummy, allowing for penetration from behind. This gives both lovers closeness while keeping still during the process.

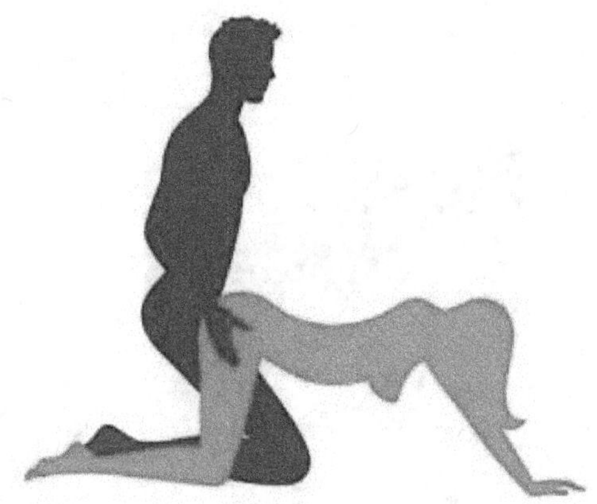

3. *Standing against the wall, then squatting.* This position allows the man to enter from behind and gives the woman the option of "pumping" or pushing against him once he is inside. He can hold on to the waist or hips to steady himself during the penetration.

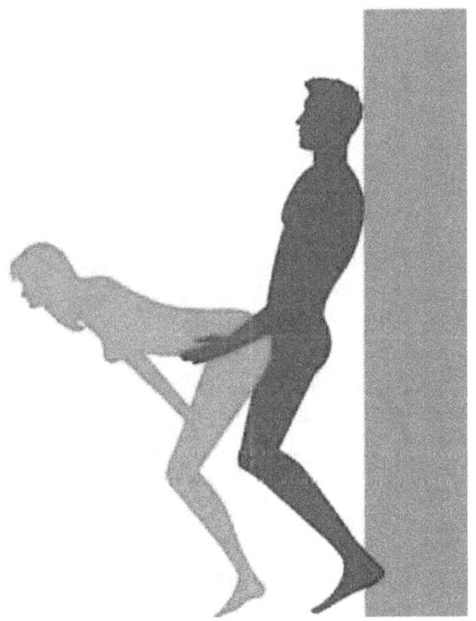

4. *Facing each other.* There is one position that allows couples to enjoy anal sex while facing each other. It involves the man sitting, legs flat and spread apart, and the woman lowering onto him, with legs on either side of his body, bent to allow better access for anal entry.

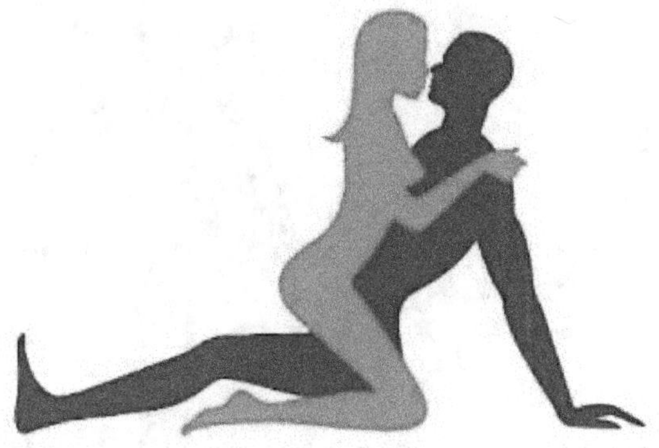

5. *Spooning.* This is another great position for anal sex, as it allows for a close, intimate touching while inside your partner. It is an ideal way to have both anal and vaginal sex.

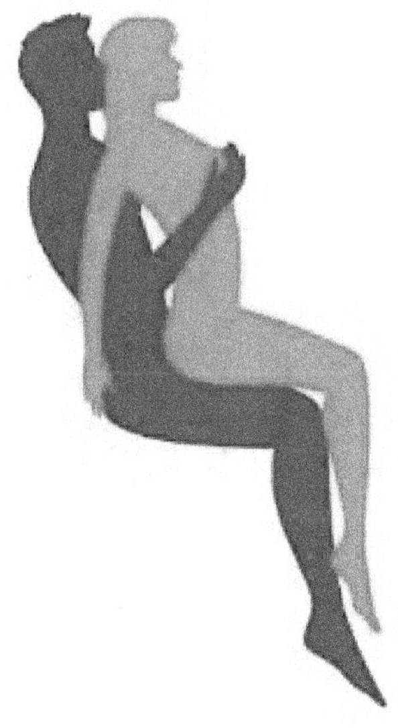

6. *The missionary position.* The missionary may not seem like a good option, though it can be if the positioning and angles are right. Lifting more and allowing for deeper penetration makes the missionary ideal for anal.

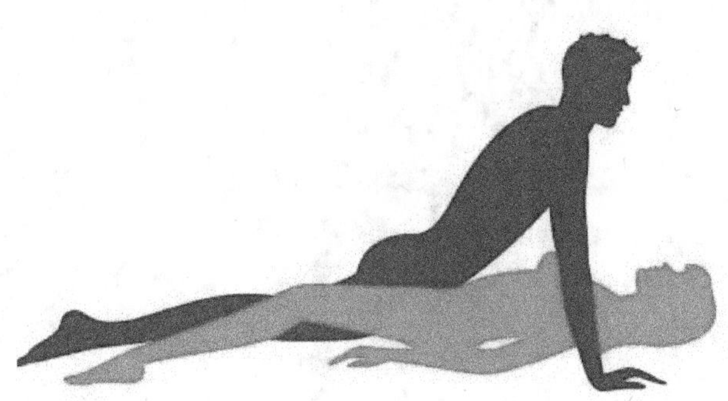

Why Is Anal Sex Pleasurable?

Most women who have had anal sex at least once consider it painful. For beginners, it can often seem like something to avoid because of the pain and initial discomfort resulting from it. For many people who handjob engage in anal sex, there is another side to this activity that involves a lot of nerve endings and pleasure, if done with patience and care, over a period of time.

Using a lot of lubrication (even more than you would normally use!) can make the experience easier to handle at first, as well as later. The sphincter is often more resistant to opening than the vagina, which makes it imperative to relax so that it can open more easily and without pain. At the opening of the anus, there is a cluster of nerve endings, which makes the experience two-fold (painful and pleasurable at the same time). The more you relax and allow slow entry, the more pleasure you will experience. On the other hand, keeping a stiff, stressed stance will not allow for entry, and further progress should stop until you feel comfortable in resuming.

Relaxing is key to successful anal sex, whether it is your first time or you have done it countless times. The anus will not open comfortably without remaining calm and with a good amount of lubrication. Using a condom is also a good idea, not only to prevent STI but also to protect the skin from friction. If you try a couple of times and feel like the experience is a failure and all your attempts at relaxing and trying different positions are to no avail, try some of the following:

Use a dildo or vibrator and a lot of lubrication. Start off with a small butt plug, and work your way to using larger sizes, closer to the size of a penis. Use as much lubrication as possible, so that you can make the most out of the experience. You can try this with your partner or solo. Some people prefer to try this alone at first so that they can be better prepared when trying anal with their partner.

Anal sex is only enjoyable if both partners are enthusiastically willing to give it a try. Some people may seem willing, but in reality, they are hesitant and will continue anyway, just to please their partner.

This should always involve mutual agreement and consent first before going beyond anyone's comfort zone.

Orgasm is achievable through anal sex for both the man and the woman. For men, the stimulation of the prostate can provide a strong orgasm, while for women, the proximity to the vagina and G-spot can have a similar effect. For people who are well acquainted with anal sex, they have learned to enjoy it for these reasons. Anal sex fits in well between other forms of sex to create a healthy, strong love life (Steig, 2019).

Chapter 12: Free Your Fantasy

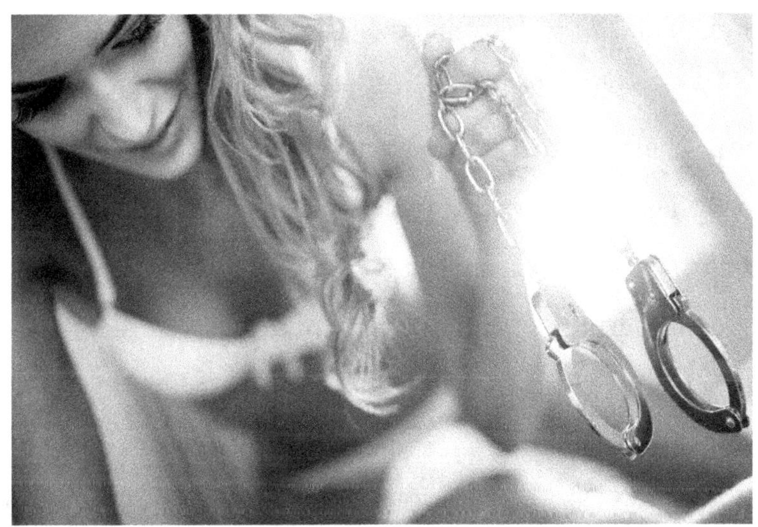

Overcoming the hurdles at the beginning of a relationship involves developing your ability to express yourself through dialogue, vocalization, and body language. This can take weeks, months, or for some people, longer, depending on personal circumstances. Once a couple becomes comfortable and open to trying new sexual experiences, many adults begin to divulge their fantasies to their partner. This can be a big step for some people who may feel embarrassed or unsure of how their partner will react to learning about secret fantasies, which may include fetishes or unique ideas that may come as a surprise.

If your partner divulges their innermost secrets about how they would like to experience pleasure, listen to them and make them feel comfortable about expressing them. If you are surprised to hear explicit details about a fetish or unexpected ideas for the bedroom, take it in stride and be attentive. Your partner will carefully observe your reaction, looking for approval and acceptance.

If their ideas disturb you or put you off, try to view from their perspective — ask questions about their fantasies and learn more about why they are drawn to trying new things. This may help you understand your partner's wants and needs better than ever.

Alternatively, expressing your own desires and fantasies can take some courage, especially if you have never discussed them with your partner or anyone else before. You may be surprised at how interested and engaged your partner is in trying something new, even if just to indulge your fantasy and give you an opportunity to feel the sensation.

Understanding the Fundamentals of BDSM

BDSM stands for bondage, dominance, submission/sadism, and masochism. It has become a popular topic in recent years with mainstream TV and films depicting aspects of this practice that are often unrealistic and inaccurate. There are many misconceptions about BDSM and whether it is harmful or pleasurable.

In general, it is a practice that can be experimented with on an occasional basis, but it can be extended into a regular event or full lifestyle.

Many people from all backgrounds in life enjoy healthy, long-term relationships that incorporate BDSM in one or more forms. Whether it is light bondage and spanking or more elaborate role-playing scenarios with specific demands and desires being met, there are many variations to customize for pleasure.

To better understand the value and enjoyment that BDSM can bring into your sex life, let us consider some facts to debunk the most common myths about this practice.

All acts performed within the context of BDSM are consensual and fully discussed at length prior to engagement. There must be full agreement and explicit consent so that all parties, whether it is a couple or more than two people involved, can experience the maximum pleasure possible.

The *submissive* is the person in a relationship or BDSM role who assumes the role of being dominated and submits to a master or dominant. Someone who takes on this position often enjoys or finds the act of submission to be sexually arousing and satisfying, as opposed to suppressing or oppressive, as some people may assume. The submissive can actually experience a sense of freedom in releasing themselves from control, allowing someone else, a trusted dominant, to relinquish that power.

The *dominant* is the person in a BDSM relationship or arrangement who plays the role of making orders or commands for their own pleasure or sexual gratification, as well as for the benefit of their "sub" or submissive. They are attentive and keen on the best interests of the submissive, even during the most intense activities, as everything is agreed upon and discussed beforehand.

A *switch* is a person who plays both the dominant and submissive roles, switching from one to another based on the scenario.

BDSM is built on a solid foundation of trust and communication. Without these key ingredients, there is no basis for a healthy BDSM relationship. In an ideal situation, the submissive signals when the session begins, when to take a break (if needed), and when they finish. A "safe word" is one way a submissive can signal to their dominant that they need a break or need to stop.

Consent is one of the most important aspects of BDSM. It must be explicit, and all parties involved must be enthusiastically willing to participate. Any sign of hesitation should be considered non-consent for the safety of the individual expressing it.

Most people who practice BDSM lead full, happy lives with families, careers and long-term marriages. It is often a misunderstood lifestyle that is wrongfully equated with abuse and mistreatment when the exact opposite is true (Wheeler, 2019).

Role-Playing and Beginning Your Journey into BDSM

Role-playing is one popular aspect of BDSM that allows partners to play the role of a dominant or submissive and as a more specific character or person. This could be as simple as dressing in a fancy dress with high heels or a tailored suit and tie. For some people, wearing a more elaborate costume to resemble a fictional character or concept is another option. Trying new roles and ideas does not have to be complex or difficult, as this would only take away from the pleasure and enjoyment of the experience. If you are looking for ideas or suggestions to begin a journey into the world of BDSM, try one of these simple recommendations:

1. Buy a beginner's kit or guide to BDSM. These are usually found in adult stores and include a few items to get you and your partner started. The items or toys are easy to use. For example, handcuffs and ties are fastened with Velcro, making it easier to remove if you don't feel comfortable at first. These kits are designed to make the transition into the lifestyle easy.

2. *Start with one technique at a time.* Get your partner involved in a dialogue about which sensations you enjoy and why. For example, you might enjoy wearing tight, restrictive garments, or perhaps you would like to experiment with a paddle or crop for spanking. If bondage is an interest, try this on its own first, and only progress once you feel comfortable doing so.

3. *Set limits and communicate often.* If you want to restrict or expand boundaries within a session, make it clear to your partner, and encourage them to do the same. Do not expect your partner to guess what you want, as this can lead to misinterpretation and may result in crossing the line.

4. *Never feel coerced.* Do not force yourself into trying a technique or practice that makes you feel uneasy or unsafe. Some people have a high threshold for pain and enjoy the sensation of a hard strike, while others are sensitive to touch and would rather scale back the intensity of a spanking or avoid it completely.

5. *Keep it light at first.* Only try more involving techniques later when you both have a basic understanding and comfort level established.

BDSM is based on trust and communication, and both of these elements are required to make it work successfully.

6. *Join a group or forum.* If you and your partner want to become acquainted with other people who practice BDSM, join a group or forum and ask questions. Explore and make new friends.

Communication is the heart and center of BDSM. Only engage in this practice with someone that you can trust, and explore with safety.

Exploring Fetishes and Kinks with Your Partner

Within the world of BDSM are many variations that go beyond the common images of bondage, whips, and blindfolds. Some people are satisfied with these activities on a mild or more progressive level, while others deviate into more niche or specific fetishes that may seem unusual or strange to the mainstream.

The most important aspect of exploring different kinks and fetishes is to ensure full and explicit consent before trying anything new.

As long as the practice is among enthusiastic, willing adults, almost anything goes and can be incorporated into play. The following fetishes go beyond the common role-play of dominant-submissive scenarios and focus entirely on objects, body parts, fashions, or other ideas that can be explored with your partner.

What is a fetish? It is a non-sexual object or concept that becomes sexualized for some people. Below are some of the most popular fetishes.

Foot Fetish

This involves a great deal of attention and care of the feet, which becomes central to the sexual experience. The mere sight of a foot or well-manicured toes can cause an immediate sexual response from someone who has a fetish for feet. Men tend to be fans of this fetish more than women. This fetish can involve many activities, from giving pedicures and massaging feet to sucking on toes and being "stepped" on as part of a dominance-submission role-playing.

Gagging or Light Choking

This is a kink that should be approached carefully to ensure that there is no harm done. Gagging should be light and easily reversed or stopped immediately if there is any discomfort at any time. Some people enjoy the sensation of being choked or gagged, which can often be done in conjunction with other forms of bondages where legs, arms, and/or the torso are confined with ties or other restraints.

Enema Play

Giving and receiving enemas is a form of pleasure for some people, and it is often used to prepare for anal play as well. The sensation of squirting water into your rectum may seem unusual if you have never tried it, as it is something only done if medically necessary. If this is something you and your partner would like to attempt, enemas can be easily found in most drug stores or pharmacies. They are sold alongside suppositories or related treatments.

Following instructions is key to prevent discomfort, and the end result can be satisfying, especially for people who enjoy administering and receiving an enema. One important thing to remember is staying close to the washroom, as enemas clear out the bowels within 5–10 minutes following administering them.

Exhibitionism and Voyeurism

These two kinks play well together and involve the enjoyment of watching (voyeurism) and being watched (exhibitionism). Voyeurism can be explored by watching your partner masturbate or by watching another couple or person engage in sexual pleasure, either in person or on film. It is important that the person or people being observed accept and consent to it, as some people are completely turned off by the idea of being watched while others will truly enjoy putting on a performance. Exhibitionism is the other side of this kink. It refers to people who are not afraid to show public displays of affection, and they go beyond when the opportunity presents itself.

Cuckolding

This fetish or kink refers to a man (or a woman) experiencing pleasure from watching their partner engage sexually with someone else, often while they observe. This can also be coupled with exhibitionism and voyeurism, as a person with the cuckolding fetish also enjoys watching their partner perform sexual acts or they enjoy being watched. Couples who are interested in this activity should ensure that condoms are used and safety precautions are taken to ensure everyone is comfortable and enthusiastic about it.

Spanking or Impact Play

Spanking or impact play is a common practice for many people involved in BDSM. They use crops, whips, or paddles to spank or "hit" their partners as part of mutual enjoyment. There is a thrill some people experience when they feel the impact of a strike to the point of sexual arousal. In some cases, striking the bottom can bring some people close to orgasm or a high level of arousal.

The most common areas of striking include the upper thighs and bottom, especially the cheeks, which can withstand a lot of striking. Even with full, explicit consent, it is best to avoid areas that can cause injury (such as the face) or anywhere there is the potential for permanent or long-term harm. Some people who practice impact play expect there to be bruises and redness. A variety of objects can be used, from light whips and floggers to canes and paddles, for a more intense impact.

Hair and Grooming Fetish

While this is not the most common fetish, it is popular in certain circles of the fetish community where hair is seen as erotic. This kink can develop in several ways, from arousal through hair cutting or shaving to long hair worship and grooming. Some people fantasize about elaborate grooming rituals that involve more than hairstyling, and it can include washing, body shaving, manicures, pedicures and specific looks or styles with hair and makeup.

The idea of involving hair as a fetish is similar to foot fetish, where regular attention is given to hair, such as brushing, playing, and tugging on it to spark arousal. This works best with a couple who enjoy this activity together. However, oftentimes one person is more engaged, while the other indulges. Scenarios may include hair salons and barbershops, capes, hairdryers, and other hair-related objects that increase arousal.

Sweater and Fur Fetish

People who become aroused by the touch or sensation of fur and soft knits or sweaters may have a fur or sweater fetish. This can be a fun experience for people who enjoy wearing such garments to turn on their partner. Some people with this fetish simply feel pleasure from watching others wear furry clothes, while others want to wear a fur coat or sweater when making love. This can be a relaxing and enjoyable fetish, as furry garments are soft and have a pleasurable texture. It is not as common as other fetishes, but it can be a fun option to explore.

Latex and Nylon

Often used with bondage, latex and nylon are materials that restrict movement when worn as garments. People who explore the sensation of nylon enjoy the sensation that this restriction involves, and they may use them on their own while pleasuring themselves or with a partner. Some people enjoy wearing garments, while others like watching other people wear certain outfits made from these garments.

There are many other kinks and fetishes to discover and explore. Some may seem more outlandish than others, but if you choose to indulge or try any of them with your partner, the key is to keep it consensual and fun (Jones, 2018).

Creating Your Own Sex Video

Sex tapes are often associated with famous celebrities and their wild sexual adventures before or during their careers. It is often the source of harsh criticism and judgment, but it is also a popular activity that many couples of all ages and backgrounds engage in. If you think the idea of a sex video is risky or taboo, there are some key items to consider before getting involved in this practice.

You will want to evaluate and consider a number of factors first. Making a video is an exciting part of a full and adventurous sex life, though it should be done with some conditions and guidelines. It is not recommended for new couples or people who do not know each other well, as there is no establishment of trust and communication may be limited or underdeveloped in the beginning. Below are some tips for couples who are considering making sex videos:

1. Discuss your ideas with your partner, and indicate that making a sex tape or video is one of them. Be direct. Let them know, and find out if they are interested in participating as well.

2. ***Do not force your partner.*** If your partner is hesitant, even for a minute, about the idea of creating a sex tape, do not push or try to convince them otherwise.

3. ***Think it over.*** If your partner approaches you about making a sex tape, explore your own internal thoughts and reactions. Consider any and all reasons for and against the making of a tape. Ask your partner their reasons as well. Don't rush into filming or decide to create your sex tape on a whim. Without some thought and consideration, you may find yourself regretting a hasty decision. It is definitely not for everyone, and it should not be regarded lightly.

4. ***Establish your limits.*** So let's say you and your partner have discussed the idea of making a sex tape in-depth, and you are excited to give it a try. There are a lot of fun and creative ways to make a sex tape while keeping some important points in mind: Some people are comfortable filming their entire body without concern, while others are self-conscious or simply uncomfortable with a full face and body view. Is there a compromise?

You might want to discuss filming parts of your body or your partner's and only within a certain part within the sexual activities. For example, you both might want to focus on recording oral sex but not anal or vaginal.

5. *Choose your scene and location.* Are you more relaxed at home in a standard bedroom setting, or would you rather try filming some action outdoors in a secluded area, such as a forest or the beach? Before you set out to find a fun outdoor space, ensure that it is a safe place to shoot, and avoid any problems, such as using a private property or a space that is not as safe (or private) as you may think.

6. *Do not forget to keep it fun and light.* Do not stress about how you or your partner look, and focus on the fun you will have off and on camera. This is a film for both of you to enjoy, and as long as you both want to enjoy it, it should be a positive experience.

7. *Make it clear from the beginning that the video you create is for your eyes only.* It should not be shared with others unless there is explicit consent to share viewing with select people or couples.

For most people, the thrill of making a sex tape gives them a rush or a thrill of being on screen. It is also a way to view and enjoy your partner on screen and in real life.

Creating a video is fun, but caution should always be taken to protect how it is stored and access to it. For many couples who enjoy filming themselves during sex, it is a way to remember their passion and to enjoy viewing later. In some extreme cases, people have shared personal videos of this nature with others outside of the relationship without prior consent. This can lead to a lot of hurt and pain, and it ruins trusting relations with your partner. Making a video should only ever be a personal experience between the couples involved.

Chapter 13: Sex Toys

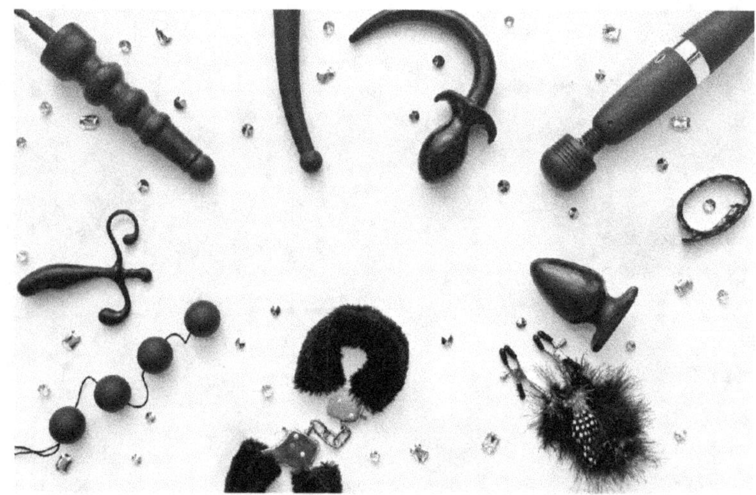

Sex toys are popular and provide an excellent means to satisfy sexual needs solo or with a partner. The days of secretly shopping for sex toys and finding them in the hidden side street shops are gone. More than ever, people are embracing their sexuality and their desire for pleasure. Toys provide an excellent way for couples to become more familiar with each other and experiment with new kinks and techniques as well.

Where to Buy Sex Toys?

Sex toys, just like pornography, were once a taboo subject, and they were only purchased from secret retailers. Fortunately, society has progressed to view sex toys and props with a positive attitude, as they can be a healthy and enjoyable way to find pleasure with your partner or on your own. There are many online and retail stores that specialize in adult toys, lingerie, and related props for a wide range of activities. To find the best options for you and your partner, consider the types of sex you want to engage in and visit a store together.

If you don't feel comfortable in a retail location, there are online stores to view many varieties of sex toys.

There are some advantages to visiting a store. You will notice other people who are interested in the same items and may feel the same way as you and partner, which will provide a sense of ease and acceptance. We often feel isolated unless we have friends that confide in us about their sexual practices. Seeing the popularity of retail stores and having the courage to enter and shop in them can make the experience more fun and enjoyable.

It is more fun and less stressful to explore items in a store. You can view many products in person and notice the actual size, texture, and features of different toys. Online descriptions for products provide details and dimensions; however, there's nothing like comparing various products together to find the right one.

Staff in adult stores are knowledgeable about the products and can answer any questions you have about how toys work and which brands or products are best for beginners to achieve certain effects and sensations.

For example, if you are new to anal sex and want to explore it, staff may suggest small butt plugs and easy lubricants to use. Online stores are convenient; however, it helps to talk to someone for more personal and customized suggestions.

If you decide to purchase products online, make sure to visit sites with your partner so that you can make the choices together based on your mutual interests and desires. It is fun to surprise your partner with a new sex toy or adventure; however, to be sure they are definitely interested, talk it over first before looking at new toys.

Sex Toys for Beginners

Deciding to buy sex toys can be fun, especially when it comes to choosing the types of toys you will test and play with. Whether you purchase online or in-person, determining which toys to choose and how they will fit into your sex life can be overwhelming at first. The following adult toys are excellent for anyone new to using them or anyone looking to try something different:

Vibrating Cock Ring

This is a great toy to get a penis erect and ready for penetration. It is also arousing for the partner, who gets to experience the sensation at the same time. This toy contains a ring that extends from a handle, where lube can be applied and keep the penis wet while it works to stimulate. It is usually under $100 and can be a fun way to take arousal to a different level.

Clitoris Vibrator

This device is a great toy for women who self-pleasure on their own or with their partner. It stimulates the clitoris, which works great during or before sex. This is an easy way to achieve clitoral stimulation on its own or as preparation for more sexual engagement.

Mini Vibrators and Eggs

These are portable, easy-to-use, and fun for couples. Small, discreet vibrators can be used anywhere, including in public, providing an unexpected amount of arousal on the go. Eggs are small egg-like vibrators that can be inserted anally for men or women to create stimulation. Before trying some adventures in public, explore first how these types of toys work for your partner and you at home. This will give you an idea of what to expect. Wear one around the house or during short trips outdoors to experiment with the sensation.

Labia and Clitoral Massagers

Like the clitoris vibrator, labia and clitoral massagers work in a similar way, only they cover more area and provide an intense experience for women.

Vibrating Butt Plugs

There are many sizes and varieties of vibrating butt plugs, from small ones for beginners to larger and longer ones with various widths and textures. For new lovers who are just starting with anal play, these are excellent to start with, as they are shaped and designed to maximize the pleasure side of anal sex with as little discomfort as possible.

Remote Control Vibrators

For couples looking to combine adventure with sex toys, these are ideal. The vibrator is inserted for play, but its vibration setting is controlled remotely, which can create an interesting scenario: one partner inserts the vibrator while the other uses the remote control. It is a fun power dynamic that allows for role-playing, especially for couples who enjoy dominant and submissive roles and exploring them further. If you play while in public, there is the effect of exhibitionism without anyone else knowing exactly what's going on, which is a thrill in itself. Remote control vibrators are great for solo play or couples alike, and as they become more popular, there are a variety of shapes and sizes to suit individual preferences and their effects.

Once you get familiar with these sex toys, you can try a variety of other options, including strap-on devices, which allow one partner to wear a dildo. This can work well with role reversal scenarios and dominance-submissive role-playing. Trying a variety of sex toys can enhance your sex life and help you achieve orgasm in different ways you may not have considered.

It can also give you a boost where there may be challenges in achieving climax for you or your partner.

Cleaning and Maintenance of Sex Toys

Deciding to buy sex toys can be fun, especially when it comes to choosing the types of toys you will test and play. It is important to take proper care of them to limit the number of bacteria and chances of infection or spreading STIs. While it is not common, if you and your partner decide to share sex toys with people or couples outside of your relationship for mutual exploration, it is best to use condoms and take their use seriously. Once you are done with your toys, it is important to clean them thoroughly, and not just with soap and water. Disinfect them by soaking in hot (boiling) water to lower any chances of bacteria. When sex toys are cleaned, store them in a dry, secure place to avoid exposure to dirt and debris. It is a good idea to clean them again soon before their use.

Once you get familiar with one or two sex toys, you may want to explore more or find new and fun ways to use them.

The world of adult play and toys is unlimited, with new versions designed to maximize pleasure being introduced on a regular basis. Many brands are designed by women for women, and likewise for men, which makes the experience closer to what we want and look for.

Chapter 14: Tricks and Tips

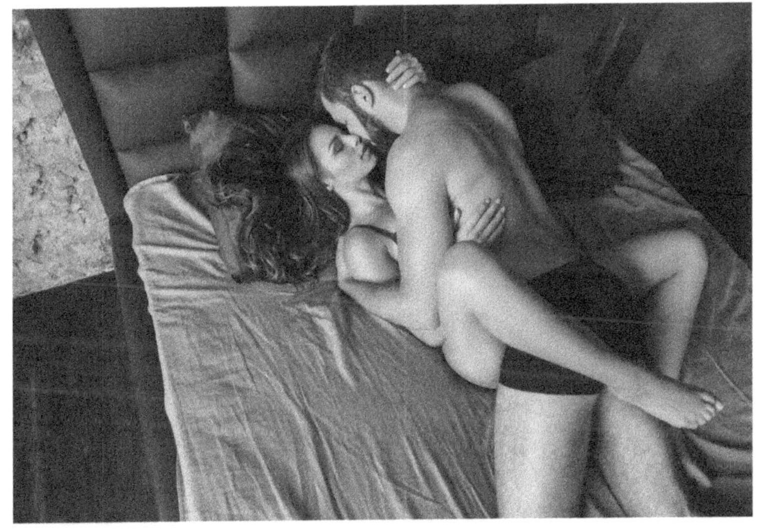

Sex does not have to become monotonous or dull, even if you have been married for many years or have a long-term partner. There are always new and exciting ways to make love and experience a new fetish or kink in the process. Many people do not realize how their sex life can expand to introduce thrilling ideas and ways of arousal you can only discover with an open mind and a sense of adventure.

It is easy to get stuck in a rut when life, work, and family become a standard routine with little room for deviation from the regular. Making an extra space of time for you and your partner becomes increasingly more important over time, as you grow more familiar and comfortable with each other. Sometimes all it takes is some imagination and a willingness to try new things without reservation. Finding the time to try new techniques can be challenging at times but worthwhile in the long term.

Frequently Asked Questions

Question: *What if my partner is not interested in exploring new aspects of intimacy with me?*

Answer: Everybody has different desires, and while couples can share a lot of things in common, there are instances where this is not the case. If you find yourself in a situation where you are interested in a specific activity or play scenario, approach the idea carefully with your spouse, especially if you are not sure how they will respond. Sometimes they may surprise you, and in other circumstances, they may not be as open. If this happens, try to offer something in exchange, and see if they are willing to try a "trade." Alternatively, simply leave it and try another technique. In reality, there are some techniques that just don't work with some couples, and skipping them completely can be the best option.

***

Question: *My partner asked if I would try anal sex, but I'm not sure it is for me.*

I'm willing to give it a try, but I'm afraid of disappointing him and not enjoying the experience. What should I do?

Answer: It is completely up to you if you want to try anal play at all, but if you do, make sure your partner understands the importance of patience and taking time to ease into it. True enjoyment for both parties results when they are content, relaxed, and ready. If there is any hesitation on your part, let him know; otherwise, take it slow and try some sex toys to get your body ready.

***

Question: *Oral sex is amazing. I wished my partner would get more involved in it, but I do not want to push him into anything he does not want to do. How can I convince him to get more involved, and is there anything I can do to persuade him?*

Answer: There's nothing wrong with a little persuasion on his part or yours when it comes to trying more oral sex or other types of sexual activity.

If he's adamantly not interested, then it may be a good idea to find an alternative; however, if he's open to persuasion, take advantage of any opportunity to convince him without getting too pushy. Get to know what he likes, too, and offer a trade: you will indulge him if he returns the favor. This can be one solution or way to work out a plan for both of you to get the most out of the situation.

***

Question: *How can I improve your confidence to work up enough courage to try something new with my partner?*

Answer: It is important to be comfortable with something before discussing it with your partner. If you have any reservations, find out more about the techniques you want to try and get familiar with them first.

This will give you the confidence you need to approach your partner and propose some ideas. If your partner wants to try something new and wants to discuss it, this is also a good opportunity to talk about interests you may want to try as well.

***

Question: *How can you move past the awkward stage of sex?*

Answer: The beginning of any new relationship can be exciting and nervous at the same time. It can take time to become acquainted with the sexual dynamic between you and your partner. Most people expect everything to unfold smoothly, but there can be some socially awkward moments even in a relationship. Keeping the lines of communication open is important in developing a strong understanding and bond with your partner. This will ease the sense of awkwardness and give you more incentive to share more together.

***

Question: *What is the secret of a long and successful sex life with your spouse or partner?*

Answer: There is no magic pill or secret to unlocking in order to find the most out of your sex life. Everything in a relationship requires a strong level of communication to know your partner and understand what's important to them.

Each relationship has its challenges; however, a lot of reasons stem from avoiding dialogue, and sometimes we make assumptions about whether we understand our partner, which can lead to misunderstandings later. Keeping the dialogue open, even when it is uncomfortable, can make life easier in the long term when we can understand each other better, and it makes intimacy more fulfilling as well. Trying new techniques and pleasing your partner are both important, and it is important that this works both ways and each person gets the most out of their enjoyment with each other.

Keeping the lines of communication open can be challenging through difficult times, and when this happens, consulting with someone you and your partner trust, such as a counselor, can be invaluable and make the hurdles easier to endure. In some cases, intimacy can take a "back seat" to life when there's too much occurring, and this can be difficult to reestablish at a later time.

Until that happens, it is important to express your feelings with your partner so that you can both be a support system for each other for years, and this is how you can overcome a lot of difficulties in life as well.

***

Question: Sometimes there are cultural and traditional differences between couples that make trying new sex techniques a challenge. How can a couple overcome this to be able to enjoy intimacy and explore new ideas?

Answer: It is never easy to explore a new idea or interest in your love life if cultural ideals or traditions you are raised with restrict sexual openness. This can be especially difficult for women when they are taught or raised to avoid discussion around sexual topics, when their sexual education is limited, and when their ideas and wants are not taken into consideration as well as they should be. Some men can feel apprehensive about trying new techniques, especially when there is a misinterpretation about them or when they feel as though they will be seen as odd or unnatural as a result.

The best way to handle these hurdles is to recognize that while it is difficult to speak about certain sexual activities, it can be worth the risk. Make sure you feel comfortable enough with your partner to express how you feel first, and try the following tips:

1. Locate a quiet, private space (e.g., a place at home where both of you can be alone) or somewhere away from home (e.g., a resort during a vacation or a retreat).

2. Rehearse what you are going to say, and make yourself as clear as possible. Begin with some positive feelings you have about your relationship with your partner, and make sure they understand that you have the best intentions in mind.

3. Ask them what they are open to trying before revealing some of your own ideas to see if they are receptive to new ideas and techniques. This can make a big difference in how well the conversation will flow. You may be pleasantly surprised to learn about how people's desires

will surface when they are given a safe and trusting environment to do so.

4. Reassure your partner that the conversation is confidential and will not leave the room, nor will it be divulged to anyone else. This type of reassurance will go a long way toward building a strong level of trust with your partner for future conversations that are delicate or private in nature. Some people do not divulge much to their partner out of fear that their partner might reveal the conversation with friends and family members who might judge them harshly or disapprove. Ensuring there is a strong level of trust in your relationship is one of the most important aspects of a successful and long-term marriage.

5. If your ideas are met with hesitation or a negative response, keep in mind that you can always try again another time without being pushy or unreasonable. Some people do not take new ideas or interests well, especially if they feel

if it conflicts with their own beliefs and perceptions. In this case, tread slowly and do not take it personally, even if it feels this way. Sometimes timing is everything, or it is how we broach the subject, not what we have to say, that makes the biggest difference.

6. Be patient and recognize that not everything is successful the first time. Don't give up. Continue to keep the lines of communication open.

***

Question: *Roleplaying seems exciting, and my partner and I are interested in exploring this, but we are new to BDSM. Before we get into any long sessions involving a few kinks, how should we start, and which toys and/or props would be suggested?*

Answer: If you and your partner are new to the world of BDSM, there are a lot of beginner kits and ideas to try before delving into more involving role-plays and sessions. First of all, keep the session brief, and focus on one technique, such as dressing up or trying a light form of bondage, for example.

If the idea of being tied up excites you and seems intimidating at the same time, try Velcro straps and ties to start. This gives beginners a sense of relief if they decide to stop or release themselves from the straps at any point during a session. Other methods to try for the first time include the following:

1. Dressing up as a character: This can be a great way to explore some of your acting abilities while impressing your partner with some creativity. For example, you might want to dress up as a fictional character or wear more fetish-style clothing, which can be found in a variety of adult and lingerie shops. Leather, corsets, and themed outfits are fun to try. Corsets can take some practice, though some people enjoy them for a variety of reasons.

2. Playing dominant and submissive roles: If you like the idea of dominant and submissive roles, try a role-play scenario that incorporates this dynamic. You may also try switching roles (letting the more dominant partner in the relationship submit instead). If you both feel

comfortable exploring this play during a short, brief encounter, try a longer session next time and add in some new activities that both of you enjoy.

3. Using paddles and canes: This may seem intimidating at first, even if they spark interest. Take it slow and try a lighter version of this kink with a beginner's kit. A light crop or whip that doesn't leave any marks but produces a thrill is a great start. Trying a lighter version is a good way to determine whether or not this activity is for you.

4. Blindfolds and experimenting with different sensations and textures: This is a mellow way to indulge in BDSM. This can involve playing with soft, furry clothes or toys that can produce a sensual response. Some sex toys have attachments or "tails" of faux fur or similar extensions that can produce a sensation while using them. Wearing furry leg warmers or

leather boots can produce a fun visual for couples.

***

Question: *Some people incorporate food into intimate play (e.g., whipped cream or fruits). Is this safe, and is there a healthy way to try it?*

Answer: Whipped cream is one of the most popular foods used during sex and foreplay. It can be used during oral play or as a way to create a trail from one part of the body to another, allowing one partner to pleasure their lover with the cream. Fruits can also be used. However, it is important to use precaution when using objects (food or non-food) that are not designed for sexual pleasure. Here are some reminders:

1. Never insert fruit, as it can cause some undesired results or reactions. Instead, use the fruit to glide against the shaft of the penis or clitoris to create arousal. Bananas are an excellent choice, as they have a silky texture that can work well against the skin.

2. Avoid any foods that you or your partner may be allergic to. Even if they are not consumed,

they could cause irritation if rubbed against your body or used during play. Examples are foods containing certain dyes or artificial flavors, as well as foods that include common allergens, such as whole wheat or gluten.

3. Try foods with a variety of textures, such as kiwis (it has soft, fuzzy peeling), peaches, and bananas. Having a variety of foods can be fun for both pleasure and snacking once you have a chance to relax afterward.

4. Wash and disinfect your foods before using them as you normally would for eating. Avoid taking any risks associated with contamination even if it seems safe. Always play in clean and comfortable spaces to minimize any problems that may arise.

5. Chocolate sauce and syrups can be fun; however, care should be taken to ensure they are not too hot (if heated). Maple syrup and honey are great options, as well as some types of jelly or pudding desserts.

***

Question: *Sometimes my partner is hard to read. I don't know if she is interested in trying or she is just doing it to please me. It can be frustrating, as I want to try new lovemaking techniques, but I don't want to push or force my ideas on someone I love. How can I find out without hurting her feelings, and how can I let her know that I accept her decision either way?*

Answer: The best way to determine how your partner truly feels is to communicate. Never proceed with any activity without your partner's explicit agreement to do so. If she agrees and you still doubt her interest, then stop until there is more conversation. There are many reasons why someone could be hesitant about the way they react or why they are afraid to speak up quickly about something they like or dislike.

If you are in a new relationship, there may be a lot to learn about your partner that they may or may not wish to divulge until they feel more comfortable. Consider the following points when approaching your spouse about engaging in sexual or intimate encounters:

1. Does your partner generally hesitate and/or change their mind often? If so, do they provide the reasons why or simply avoid further discussion? If they are not willing to talk about it or are prone to sudden changing of the mind, slow down significantly or stop completely. Do not risk any unnecessary harm, even if unintentional. Talk about it first.

2. Are you aware of any traumatic experiences in the past or situations that your partner may have experienced that could have an impact on their ability to enjoy intimacy? If your marriage or relationship is new, there may be less you know about them. It is not something you should take personally, as many people who have endured traumatic events, including abuse, may not speak about it at all, including to those who love them most.

3. Determine your partner's "hard" and "soft" limits. This is a practice used in BDSM. A "hard" limit means it is a definite no, while a "soft"

limit indicates a possibility to explore, although maybe not immediately. Some things take time, and establishing boundaries is the most important way to know where your partner is willing to go and when they need to stop.

4. Some people are just not good at talking about their feelings or thoughts. When this happens, it can be difficult to get to know someone despite your best efforts. This may change in time when comfort levels improve. However, it still remains vital to communicate even when the other person does not respond. It lets them know that you care and you are willing to help and support them. Keep it up, and they will eventually open to conversation.

5. Finally, your partner is responsible for communicating, too, and if you have done your part, it is up to them. Patience is key. Sometimes helping someone else to find the right words or things to say can be challenging. Not everyone is

good at finding their way to communicate even if they want to.

***

Question: My partner has insecurities about his body. How can I help him overcome these insecurities?

Answer: One of the most powerful ways you can show support to your partner is by communicating your acceptance of them and their bodies. Sometimes, our bodies change, and this can impact how we respond to each other in a relationship. If there are health reasons that negatively affect your partner's physical appearance, showing support is the best way to help them through difficult times. Show them affection even if it does not lead to sex or intimacy, and assure them they are desired. This will go a long way to build their sense of security and help them cope with their situation.

Some people struggle with diet and improving their physical shape, which can definitely impact their love life. Making critical remarks, even if they are considered constructive, can be discouraging.

If your partner is making strides toward improvement, join them and be the best support system they have. Your support and acceptance are most vital to your partner, especially during challenging times when they may doubt their own ability to achieve success. Take morning walks or cycling trips with them, and make better dietary choices together. View it as a partnership in this sense, where your partner's challenges are also yours, and help them to conquer their fears and achieve their goals. Not only will the result improve your life together, but it will also improve your intimacy and closeness for years.

Conclusion

Intimacy is an important part of a healthy relationship, and people's sexual needs change and evolve over time. Some couples are eager to experiment and try new techniques early in the relationship, while others are more reserved. Other couples or individuals may explore outside of their comfort zone or regular boundaries for something less conventional later in life. The way we are raised and society's view on the idea of intimacy can play a major role in influencing how we approach love, sex, and relationships. Fortunately, society has grown more accepting of a more open approach to sex and intimacy, making it easier for more people to talk candidly and comfortably about their desires and ideas.

Sometimes a small change, such as a minor adjustment in a position or a new style of oral sex, can make a tremendous boost in your sex life.

Exploring something a bit different — such as a new setting, technique, or just the discussion of an idea (as subtle or wild as it may be) — can make a profound improvement in how we engage with our partner. Never underestimate the power of a simple suggestion or shared thought, even if done on a whim. If your partner shares their ideas with you, consider this as a new opportunity of fun you can explore with them or, at the very least, a good start toward communicating about your shared experiences and needs. Displaying a willingness and having a partner who is on board with exploring many options is what an ideal relationship strives for. While communication and trust are the foundation of a successful relationship and intimacy, learning to accept new and exciting experiences can make a major improvement in your love life.

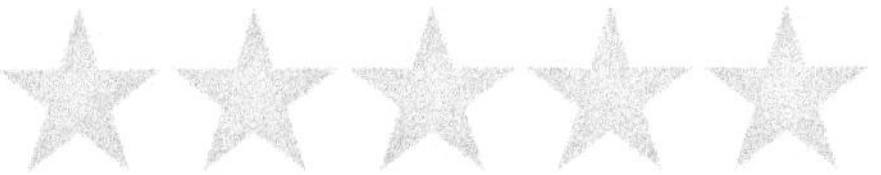

We hope you enjoyed this title.
For us, there is no greater reward
than your satisfaction.

If you liked this book, please leave
a review.

References

Carson, T. (2017). 6 weird things you didn't know about sex. Retrieved from https://www.hercampus.com/wellness/sexual-health/6-weird-things-you-didn-t-know-about-sex

Eliason, N. (n.d.). The best sex positions for multiple orgasms for men. Retrieved from https://www.nateliason.com/blog/multiple-orgasms-sex-men

Emery, L. R. (2018). Retrieved from https://www.bustle.com/p/the-best-sex-positions-that-seem-weird-but-are-actually-kind-of-great-7844463

Gilmour, P. (2019). Silent vibrators that let you orgasm in peace. Retrieved from https://www.cosmopolitan.com/uk/love-sex/sex/g13462217/quiet-silent-sex-toys/?slide=7

Gordon, S. (2018). 20 things we all need to know about sex. Retrieved from https://www.iol.co.za/lifestyle/love-sex/sex/20-things-we-all-need-to-know-about-sex-11329888

Hubby, K. (2017). The most bizarre facts about sex you should probably know. Retrieved from https://www.dailydot.com/irl/sex-facts/

James, J. (n.d.). The best ways to jerk off: 20 awesome male masturbation techniques to cum like a champ! Retrieved from https://www.menstoyshub.com/male-masturbation-techniques

Jameson, S. (n.d.) 28 incredible anal sex positions (with pictures!) for wild, orgasmic sex. Retrieved from https://badgirlsbible.com/anal-sex-positions

Jameson, S. (n.d.). 14 powerful masturbation techniques for incredible orgasms. Retrieved from https://badgirlsbible.com/masturbation-techniques

Klepchukova, A. (2019). How to achieve vaginal orgasm: 9 unforgettable tips. Retrieved from https://flo.health/menstrual-cycle/sex/pleasure/how-to-achieve-vaginal-orgasm

Krisher, H. (n.d.) Retrieved from https://www.webmd.com/sex-relationships/features/7-awesome-erogenous-zones#1

Marin, V. (2016). 8 ways to seduce your man or woman when you're in a longterm relationship. Retrieved from https://www.bustle.com/articles/96817-8-ways-to-seduce-your-man-or-woman-when-youre-in-a-longterm-relationship

REL Rules. (n.d.). 13 common mistakes people make during sex. Retrieved from https://relrules.com/13-common-mistakes-people-make-during-sex/

Relationship Guide Review (2019). Retrieved from https://relationshipguidesreview.com/how-to-overcome-shyness-in-bed/

Scaccia, A. (2018). Retrieved from https://www.healthline.com/health/healthy-sex/tantric-sex#how-to-prepare-your-mind

Steig, C. (2019). Why anal sex is pleasurable for some people — but not everyone. Retrieved from https://www.refinery29.com/en-us/does-anal-sex-feel-good

Surnow, R. (2016). Tantric sex. Retrieved from https://www.cosmopolitan.com/sexopedia/a8100798/how-to-have-tantric-sex/

Thomas, S. (2017). Here's what you need to know about fisting. Retrieved from https://www.refinery29.com/en-us/what-is-fisting

Wheeler, G. (2019). What is BDSM? A sex expert reveals exactly what it means. Retrieved from https://www.elitedaily.com/p/what-is-bdsm-a-sex-expert-reveals-exactly-what-it-means-8068256